CHEKHOV'S DOCTORS

Literature and Medicine
MARTIN KOHN AND CAROL DONLEY, EDITORS

Chekhov's Doctors

A Collection of

Chekhov's Medical Tales

Edited by Jack Coulehan

Foreword by Robert Coles

The Kent State

University Press

KENT & LONDON

© 2003 by The Kent State University Press, Kent, Ohio 44242
Library of Congress Catalog Card Number 2003012902
ISBN 0-87338-780-5
Manufactured in the United States of America

Grateful acknowledgment for permission to use the following:

"An Unpleasantness" from *The Unknown Chekhov: Stories and Other Writings*,
trans. Avram Yarmolinsky. Translation copyright © 1954 Avram Yarmolinsky.
Copyright renewed 1982 Babette Deutsch Yarmolinsky.
Reprinted by permission of Farrar, Straus and Giroux, LLC.

"Intrigues" from *The Undiscovered Chekhov: Forty-three New Stories*,
trans. Peter Constantine. Reprinted by permission of Seven Stories Press.

07 06 05 04 03   5 4 3 2 1

Library of Congress Cataloging-in-Publication Data
Chekhov, Anton Pavlovich, 1860–1904.
[Short stories. English. Selections]
Chekhov's doctors : a collection of Chekhov's medical tales /
Jack Coulehan, editor ; foreword by Robert Coles.
p.   cm.—(Literature and medicine ; 5)
Includes bibliographical references.
ISBN 0-87338-780-5 (alk. paper)
1. Chekhov, Anton Pavlovich, 1860–1904—Translations into English. 2. Physicians—
Fiction. I. Coulehan, John L., 1943– II. Title. III. Literature and medicine (Kent, Ohio) ; 5.
PG3456.A13C68 2003
891.73'3—dc21   2003012902

British Library Cataloging-in-Publication data are available.

If a great many remedies
are suggested for some disease,
it means the disease is incurable.
　　　—THE CHERRY ORCHARD

The end of the century
has come upon us
without a sign of release
or the beginning of justice.
We're selling the orchard
to pay our debts
and reminiscing about
love's excitements,
life's mistakes. I suspect
a century ago the hearts
of the people sitting here
were just as generous,
intense, and cruel as ours.

A miniature flower
thrives in the moisture
and dust of a broken
pavement—this is the gist
of the matter. We want
so strongly to believe
the flower will spread
everywhere. How quickly
it dies! If the disease
had a cure, we would not need
so many remedies.
　　　—JACK COULEHAN

Contents

Foreword to Chekhov's Doctors

ROBERT COLES

What follows are stories by a writer who was also a physician—tales of sadness and woe, but also of surprise and hope, all of them meant to remind the reader of various aspects of human nature: the possibilities for the good and bad that await expression in our individual lifetimes. Anton Chekhov has been dead almost a century and lived a relatively short life of forty-four years (like Orwell's and D. H. Lawrence's, his writing life was cut short by tuberculosis). Yet, in the brief time fate gave him, the Russian doctor, a serf's grandson, wrote short and longer fiction; he also attended the world as an observer and became a documentary essayist; and not least, he became a much admired dramatist, whose plays continue to engage and inspire theatergoers. As is the case with his predecessor, Dostoievsky, and his older friend, Tolstoy, Chekhov remains a nineteenth-century Russian giant whose words continue to offer readers the world over penetrating moral and psychological contemplation.

Needless to say, our finest writers speak in many voices and are heard by listeners (readers) who have their own inclinations and interests—hence the broad range of interpretive responses granted the imaginative narrative work of Chekhov. In a sense, this book is one such reply—on the part of a doctor–reader (and poet) to the doctor stories of a doctor–writer. An American physician gives much thought to a Russian physician's extraordinary work, accomplished long ago—though the latter is still very much an ethically prodding presence among us who want to ask ourselves the big questions that the stories ahead beg us to consider: the meaning and purpose of life, and the manner it ought to be conducted (and why).

In his helpful and quite instructive introduction, our present-day Dr. C. tells us much about the Dr. C. whose stories we are to read—and inevitably, about the constraints that bear on a writer who wants to get at the heart of the matter for his readers. Here, then, are some chosen tales, all of which have a doctor in them: in their sum, they are medical protagonists, each trying to find a way toward honor and decent living, and each not altogether sure that such an achievement has been securely obtained. Put differently, Chekhov wanted, for those doctors he rendered, a confrontation that would disclose the truth of their moral (and spiritual) lives; he has accidents and incidents befall them, and the outcome stirs us to consider ourselves—who we are, what we hold dear, and what we will all too willingly forego (the loyalties and obligations we might set aside with an abandon, and at a price, under certain circumstances). Through a writer's talent, the writer's way of letting things happen in the plot unfolded, we may indeed squirm as we learn of the substantial squirming that occurs in the Chekhovian tales of professional obligation and duty and become, commonly, the victims of an enveloping and overweening ambition and pride (all of that moral drama a latter-day echo of the message offered long ago by well-known Greek playwrights, in whose company the author of *Uncle Vanya, The Three Sisters,* and *The Cherry Orchard* very much belongs).

Again and again Chekhov presents us with doctors summoned not only by their patients, but by the taxing, even overwhelming personal challenges (and problems) that threaten them severely, even as they try (sometimes with eventual success, sometimes in vain) to do their work, make their home visits, and speak with some goodness of mind and heart. These doctors frequently fall flat on their faces—become themselves the sick and troubled ones whom we know no profession, class, or race lacks in significant numbers. In the longest story ahead (a novella really) Chekhov gives us "Ward No. 6" whose physician is soon enough a psychological (and moral) compatriot of the patients with whom he is entrusted. Chekhov wants to blur lines all too readily and conventionally upheld. A doctor who is involved in the clinical life of a hospital begins to enjoy conversing with patients, rather than medicating them casually, by rote—soon enough earns the perplexity of others, then their remove. An attending physician has become a strange one, not unlike those others on Ward Six—a writer's gradually constructed assertion that an illness, even a psychiatric one, can step by step become catching.

In "A Nervous Breakdown," we are asked to go further in that direction, consider the manner in which some of us doctors "treat" those who don't quite fit in socially, don't react in the usual or customary way—their moral sensitivity prompts them to dismay, even horror, at the sight of the world's cruelty, hurt, and suffering, whereas so-called normal people, the "well adjusted," shrug their shoulders through indifference or even bemusement, in the face of such injustice and human pain. Chekhov has a medical student, an artist, and a law student together go visit a neighborhood of brothels. Only the law student is moved to moral concern, to sympathy for those exploited by individuals anxious to serve their bodily appetites, with no regard for the price paid by others, all too categorically dismissed as "prostitutes" (such labels a form of self-serving blindness). The law student becomes exceedingly upset; he goes through what the story's title forecasts, "a nervous breakdown"—and the medical student, alas, wants a doctor's treatment for Vassilyev, the law student, whose words of inwardness, of observation and reflection, have so very much to tell us: "That I should have taken my degree in two faculties," Chekhov has him to say to Mayer, the medical student, "You look upon as a great achievement." Then, to strengthen what will become a powerful moral aside: "Because I have written a work which in three years will be thrown aside and forgotten, I am praised up to the skies; but because I cannot speak of fallen women as unconcernedly as of these chairs, I am being examined by doctors, I am called mad, and I am pitied."

Each of us, of course, will find his or her Chekhovian moment—though arguably, right there (in that charged critique of so very much that is cultural and political), a writer takes on for all of us the matter of moral freedom: what we yield of ourselves to others to go along with the status quo—unless, like the law student, we dare have our ethically prompted say. Put otherwise, Chekhov dared remind himself, and his medical colleagues, that doctors can become the all too willing agents of social conformity, the agents, too, of persecutions, as Russia's and China's doctors of our time vividly have shown us to be possible and may sometimes be the case elsewhere, even on turf close to us who read these stories.

Chekhov in the previous passage moved toward philosophical and ideological terrain and indeed literally ventured into similar territory—the Sakhalin Island, off the coast of Siberia, that had become a vast penal colony, a place of indignity, of severe and arbitrary punishment, and of state-sponsored persecution. To get to his destination, this earnestly compassionate, morally awake doctor, already ailing with the tuberculosis that would cause his death, had to travel long and hard—the voyage a threat to a life quite fragile, even endangered. But go he did, and the result was a "doctor's visit" other than the one described in the namesake story. In *The Island of Sakhalin* (1895), Chekhov became a writer of travel, of firsthand social observation, of the documentary effort and essay that becomes an instrument of political thinking—a society closely watched through the lives of its troubled and hardened and altogether vulnerable ones, locked up at distance, but now brought to the reading notice of an audience (in Moscow and St. Petersburg) a continent away. A highly esteemed teller of stories had shifted his field of sight and responsive narrative exertion into an altogether new realm—from villages with the meek and the mighty, tenuously yet constantly engaged, to prisons and those who run them, at no small moral cost to themselves. Chekhov's everpresent willingness to look wide and deep was once more accorded the life of a brilliant, knowing writer's exactly crafted words.

We are mighty lucky to have this book, courtesy of Dr. Coulehan's writerly embrace of a passionately able and inspired fellow physician whose powerfully affecting and suggestive storytelling has now been so thoughtfully made available. I only wish that two other American physicians, each of them, like Chekhov, a skillful and compelling writer of stories, were here to enjoy their Russian comrade in arms. I have in mind Dr. William Carlos Williams, whose doctor stories connect in spirit with those of Dr. Chekhov—the American doctor more intent on conveying the momentary problems of practicality in his medical office (and the consequences to patient and physician alike), and the Russian doctor eager to convey the moods that such occasions set in motion, the mix of anticipation on the other. "Read Chekhov, read story after story of his" Dr. Williams once told a medical student fortunate to know him and anxious for advice: "I turn to him [Chekhov] all the time; stories like 'Anyuta' and 'Enemies' remind me of the danger around the corner, in this doctoring life: smugness, and one of the consequences, callousness, and then the decline into being a big shot, full of oneself (the occupational hazards of our trade)—Chekhov knew of all that, saw it in others, and thereby saw himself in danger." So it was, too, Dr. Walker Percy, another American doctor–writer, a novelist of great distinction, who once ruminating on "influences" remarked: "I think of Chekhov as the deservedly revered father of all of us who have turned to the typewriter to let others know what goes on when you're dueling with death, hoping to win for the sake of your patients, and for the sake of yourself as well: Chekhov is the master of letting us all know that!" Yes, indeed—and thanks to this book, and its editor's search for Chekhov's many truths—we can stop and through our reading reflect on many matters, courtesy of an inviting reservoir of the enlightenment and wisdom, worked into stories wonderfully told and now, knowingly, gracefully assembled and presented.

Introduction

❧

1.

The postcard is a reproduction of an oil painting, a familiar and sentimental late-nineteenth-century scene—a darkened sick room with a narrow shaft of light, a doctor sitting at the foot of a child's bed, a second child playing on the floor. The doctor appears to be reassuring the anxious mother, who stands beside him, hanging on every word. The sick child stares longingly from the shadows. The barefoot woman wears crumpled clothes and a babushka. Is the news good or bad? Will the child survive? Whatever the outcome this doctor embodies the ideals of fidelity and compassion. It is a familiar domestic scene in popular art of the time, if not in reality. What makes this particular painting so unusual is the identity of the doctor—Anton Pavlovitch Chekhov, one of great masters of world literature.

The reverse side of the postcard, which I purchased at the entrance kiosk to Chekhov's estate at Melikhovo, contains a quotation from a letter to Alexei Suvorin, Chekhov's friend and editor, in which the author explains, "While you have been inviting me to Vienna . . . I have been busy being sole doctor of the Serpehovskovo district, and trying to catch cholera by the tail and organize health services. I have in my district 25 villages, 4 factories, and 1 monastery. In the morning I receive patients and in the afternoon go on house calls" (to Suvorin, August 16, 1892).

At the time he wrote the letter to Suvorin the author had recently purchased the small, dilapidated estate and moved with his family from Moscow. He was energetically renovating—planting trees, putting in a garden, and remodeling the house. However, no sooner had the Chekhovs settled at Melikhovo than a cholera epidemic threatened the region. And then there were so many sick peasants. Soon Chekhov was up and running, practicing medicine and public health by day and writing masterpieces like "The Grasshopper" and "Ward No. 6" by night.

How did he find the time and energy to pursue two such demanding careers? Several years earlier, at the height of Chekhov's early literary success, the same Alexei Suvorin had urged the young writer to give up medicine. Medicine is a waste of your time and energy, he said. Take my advice, you'd better learn to play the game. Become more focused. You'll never reach your potential unless you concentrate on writing. In response, Chekhov wrote, "You advise me not to chase after two hares at once and to forget about practicing medicine. Well, I don't see what's so impossible about chasing two hares at once. . . . Medicine is my lawful wedded wife and literature my mistress. When one gets on my nerves, I spend the night with the other. This may be somewhat disorganized, but then again it's not boring, and anyway, neither loses anything by my duplicity." In this famous passage the twenty-eight-year-old writer dances lightly over a fundamental truth of his life and identity. In fact Chekhov's career wasn't so much a matter of jumping back and forth from one bedroom to another, as was the case later perhaps with the poet Wallace Stevens or the composer Charles Ives. Rather, Chekhov thrived on the effective, if not always seamless, integration of the arts of medicine and writing, which reinforced one another throughout his creative life.

By the time young Anton graduated from the University of Moscow School of Medicine in 1884 he was already a professional writer. His affair with the muse had started innocently enough. The grandson of serfs, Anton was the third of six children in a poor merchant family from Taganrog, a provincial town deep in the south of Russia on the shore of the Sea of Azov. His stern, moralistic father fared poorly in the retail business and went bankrupt when the boy was sixteen years old. While the rest of the family moved to Moscow to seek a better future, Anton remained behind in Taganrog to finish high school. Though even then he was amusing himself by writing plays and sketches, the adolescent Chekhov decided to become a physician, perhaps influenced by the positive image projected by a Dr. Schrempf, who had treated him for peritonitis when he was fifteen. Thus in 1879 the nineteen-year-old arrived in Moscow, scholarship in hand, and began his medical studies. He also discovered his family living in squalor. His father's job paid poorly. His older brothers were irresponsible. The apartment was appalling. Anton soon discovered that he could help ameliorate the situation by selling his stories and sketches to local papers for eight kopecks per line. He wrote obsessively on nights and weekends, often knocking off a story or two in a day, ultimately publishing more than two hundred during this period, all under pseudonyms like Mr. Balastov, the Man without a Spleen, or (his preferred) Antosha Chekhonte.

These proved so successful that by the time he graduated in 1884, Anton was the acknowledged family breadwinner. However, although the student Chekhov viewed his writing pragmatically, the young physician soon came to view literature as integral to his identity. The writing appeared to come effortlessly. Whatever he saw or heard in life bubbled-up into a tale. Thus, it wasn't surprising that the newly minted Doctor Chekhov continued to write after he had hung up a shingle at his rented house in Moscow, and the patients began to arrive. "Continued to write" doesn't exactly do justice to Chekhov's productivity—he published fifty-four stories in 1885, seventy-six in 1886, and fifty-seven in 1887. During this period he garnered the notice of well-known authors and editors, especially Alexei Suvorin, the editor–owner of *New Times,* an influential St. Petersburg periodical. Soon the young writer graduated from pulp fiction into the literary elite; his advancement capped in 1888 by receiving the Pushkin Prize, one of Russia's most prestigious literary honors.

Yet Chekhov never turned away from medicine, which remained an integral part of his self-consciousness, though writing increasingly demanded the lion's share of his time. In 1889 Chekhov did, in fact, retire from "normal" practice; he never again charged for his medical services, even though he never became a wealthy man and frequently found himself strapped for money. Nonetheless, he pursued his medical identity at the expense of his writing career—by providing free care to the country folk near Melikhovo (as depicted in the painting), by donating his services to the government as a district physician, and by engaging regularly in public health initiatives. In less than five months in 1891, Chekhov reported seeing 453 patients at a district health center and making 576 house calls, in addition to his home practice. Throughout his life, Chekhov also was heavily involved in "grassroots" activism, building schools for peasants, raising funds to help famine victims, and, later, near the end of his life, supporting the establishment of a sanitarium for tuberculosis victims at Yalta.

One of the most well known of these public health efforts was his epidemiological survey of health and social conditions in the prison colonies on Sakhalin Island in 1890. Traveling by himself, Chekhov left Moscow in April 1890 and journeyed six weeks by train, steamboat, and horse-drawn carriage across Siberia to reach the 1000-kilometer-long island. There he embarked on a one-man, three-month survey of the population, tenaciously picking his way from settlement to settlement and from house to house, often by foot. Biographers have long tried to pinpoint his motivation for this perilous journey. During the year prior to the trip to Sakhalin, Chekhov had undergone a crisis of confidence. Was he a good enough writer? Was he an adequate doctor? Did he really have what it takes? What direction should he pursue in the future? In a letter to Suvorin he opined, "I don't love money enough for medicine, and I lack the necessary passion—and therefore talent—for literature. The fire in me burns with an even, lethargic flame; it never flares up or roars . . . I have very little passion. Add to that the following psychopathic trait: for two years now, seeing my works in print has for some reason given me no pleasure" (to Suvorin, May 4, 1889). These reported experiences—lack of passion and loss of pleasure—suggest that he may have had an episode of clinical depression, perhaps in part precipitated by the recent death of his brother Nicholas from tuberculosis. There were also literary issues. He had promised himself and his friends that he would turn his attention to a novel, a big book that would establish him as a truly serious writer. But he couldn't do it; the novel didn't come.

However, the overt reason for Sakhalin—as opposed to embarking on some other major project or life change—was Chekhov's desire to pay his debt to medicine. He had developed a scientific interest in penology and became aware of the Russian government's establishment of penal colonies on the distant Pacific island, which had recently been wrested from Japanese control. Although Chekhov had graduated as a medical doctor, he had never completed the research thesis (the equivalent of a Ph.D.) that would make him eligible to become a professor. Hence, his debt to medicine—he would document health status and living conditions in the prison colonies.

Ultimately, Chekhov visited every settlement and aimed to survey every household on Sakhalin, using a twelve-item data collection form for demographic and medical information. He later claimed to have completed over ten thousand of these forms in three months, a feat that (if true) qualifies Chekhov as the speediest shoe-leather epidemiologist of all time. The author found it difficult to write of his work on Sakhalin Island. What form should the writing take? He had planned to make it a scientific monograph, but the creative artist struggled with the limitations of data and inference. What about his personal experience? And what about the interesting stories he heard some of the prisoners tell? After struggling with the material for years, Chekhov published *The Island of Sakhalin* (1895), a curious (but often engrossing) mixture of geography, history, medicine, statistics, and travelogue. Unfortunately, the University of Moscow was not impressed.

In early 1892 Chekhov purchased the rundown Melikhovo estate. He and his family lived there for the next six years, his "middle period," during which he matured as a writer as well as a humanitarian. This is also the period depicted in the painting of Dr. Chekhov visiting a sick child. The thirty-something landowner of Melikhovo wrote fewer stories than he had in his youth. However, the majority of these are masterpieces, including most of his great novellas ("The Duel," "An Anonymous Story," "A Woman's Kingdom," "Three Years," and "My Life"). Here, too, he wrote his groundbreaking plays *The Seagull* and *Uncle Vanya.*

But what was this 1890s Chekhov like? Picture a middle-aged bachelor, longish face, rather neatly trimmed beard, a pince-nez clipped to the bridge of his nose. The man is a paterfamilias whose household consists of his parents and his sister Masha, a teacher who has become his confidant and secretary. His three surviving brothers look to him for guidance and sometimes for financial help. He is popular in literary circles, witty, and generous with his time and energy. Yet, too, he enjoys the solitude of his garden. The Chekhovs often entertain guests at Melikhovo, and quite commonly numbered among the guests are Anton's women admirers. His encounters with women are flirtatious and obviously enjoyable. Over the years he conducts teasing, sexually charged relationships (largely by letter) with several women, especially Lika Mizinova, a teacher-friend of Masha's. Whether any of these liaisons are "affairs" is uncertain. Most biographers conclude that Chekhov's emotional reserve and ambivalence about commitment kept these friendships from being consummated. Hence, the teasing and tension remained nonphysical. More recently, Donald Rayfield in his massive biography *Anton Chekhov* suggests that the author's "stringing along" was doubly cruel because it concealed a series of true sexual relationships. Nonetheless, the Chekhov of Melikhovo remains a bachelor.

The doctor in the painting already suffers from the tuberculosis that will kill him at the age of forty-four years. In fact he had first coughed blood when he was still a medical student. Yet Chekhov dismissed that episode and each subsequent episode over many years as "influenza" or "bronchitis," steadfastly refusing to give himself the diagnosis of consumption. As a physician Chekhov surely must have been aware of the meaning of his symptoms, especially during the period when he spent weeks nursing his brother Nicholas, who died of tuberculosis in 1889. Was Chekhov aware that he suffered from tuberculosis, but simply chose to deny it to others? Or was this a case of such massive denial that the man did not understand his own condition? The cat was finally let out of the bag in early 1897. While dining at a restaurant in Moscow, Chekhov suddenly experienced a violent spell of hemoptysis (coughing blood) that left him critically ill. He was admitted for the first time to a medical clinic, in fact, a clinic run by Dr. Ostropov, one of his medical school professors. After this episode, Chekhov's illness resulted in progressive physical limitation, and he was no longer able to deny its nature. Weakness, coughing, and shortness of breath defined his life. At the insistence of his doctors Chekhov left his beloved Melikhovo and spent much of the year at his new home in the sunny Black Sea resort of Yalta.

It was also during these last years that the bachelor writer courted and married Olga Knipper, an actress with the Moscow Theater Arts Company. Even after their marriage in 1901 Olga remained at work in Moscow during much of the year, while the invalid Chekhov lived in Yalta. He found himself able to devote less and less of his waning energy to writing, especially because he refused to give up his many social and philanthropic activities. Nonetheless, between 1898 and his death in 1904 Chekhov completed some of his greatest work, including several stories, two novellas ("Peasants" [1897] and "In the Ravine" [1900]), and his last plays, *The Three Sisters* (1900) and *The Cherry Orchard* (1903).

2.

In Chekhov's story "About Love" (1898), the narrator speculates on the nature of love. What is its essence? What are universal characteristics that identify love wherever it occurs? "What seems to fit one instance doesn't fit a dozen others," the narrator concludes. "It's best to interpret each instance separately in my view, without trying to generalize. We must isolate each individual case, as doctors say." Indeed, Chekhov's stories and plays rigorously follow this dictum. While many of his Russian contemporaries used fiction to advance their moral or social theories, Dr. Chekhov focused on the complexities of human interaction. In Chekhov's world, biology and circumstance constrain human freedom. People don't listen to one another. Communication often fails. Acts performed with good intentions frequently result in hurtful outcomes. Yet occasionally and in unexpected places, one finds a glimmer of love, courage, spirituality, or healing. "Never generalize," Chekhov tells his readers. "Never theorize. Pay attention to the particulars. Focus on the concrete." In this respect, the nineteenth-century physician–storyteller presages the twentieth-century physician–poet, William Carlos Williams, who coined the aphorism, "No ideas but in things."

Chekhov experienced no conflict between art and science, or art and medicine. He believed that knowledge of one complements the other. He explained this to Suvorin: "If a man knows the theory of the circulatory system, he is rich. If he learns the history of religion and the song 'I Remember a Marvelous Moment' in addition, he is the richer, not the poorer for it. We are consequently dealing entirely in pluses" (to Suvorin, May 15, 1890). In an 1899 autobiographical statement prepared for his medical school classmate the neurologist Dr. Grigory Rossolimo, Chekhov confirmed that his clinical "eye" and medical knowledge are important characteristics of his writing: "My knowledge of natural sciences and scientific methods has made me careful and I have always tried, when possible, to take into consideration the scientific data. When it was not possible, I preferred not to write at all" (to Rossolimo, Oct. 11, 1899).

Chekhov brought medical knowledge and sensitivity to his creative writing. Several characteristics of his work reveal the influence of medical training. For example, he used his medical knowledge to lend accuracy to descriptions of diseases and medical situations. This characteristic is perhaps most clearly seen in Chekhov's description of mental disorders. For example, the title character in *Ivanov*, Chekhov's first full-length play, is a subtle portrait of a man suffering from clinical depression, who eventually commits suicide. The young heiress in "A Doctor's Visit" (included in this collection) presents symptoms we would now label generalized anxiety or panic disorder. The title character in *Uncle Vanya* appears to have characterologic or constitutional depression, which today we would likely call "dysthymia." In the peculiar story called "The Black Monk," Chekhov describes a psychotic condition, presumably schizophrenia. As we see, the author's intimate knowledge of medicine and medical practice also allowed him to create numerous physician characters at work in clinical or public health environments.

However, medical attitudes and methodology play a far larger role in Chekhov's work than does specific medical knowledge. He believed that his duty as a writer was to present his observations clearly and accurately; in other words, to lay out the data in an objective fashion and allow readers to reach their own conclusions, rather than provide an author's interpretation. He wrote, "The artist should not be a judge of his characters and what they say, but only an objective observer" (to Suvorin, May 30, 1888).

Chekhov's commitment to introducing the objectivity of science into his writing was a source of conflict with Tolstoy, at that time Russia's most beloved writer, widely revered as a living saint. The two men enjoyed a close personal bond despite the great difference in their ages, but they approached writing (and living) with radically different philosophies. After his midlife religious conversion, Tolstoy viewed literature as a way to communicate his moral vision. He preached the gospel of a radical Christianity, in which all men (but certainly not women—Tolstoy was a thoroughgoing misogynist) would achieve economic and social equality. However, Tolstoy rejected material progress. He did not believe that the fruits of science could benefit mankind; in particular, he was skeptical of medicine and doctors. He said that Chekhov would be a better writer if he gave up medicine. Chekhov, on the other hand, complained, "Tolstoy calls doctors scoundrels and flaunts his ignorance of important matters because he is a second Diogenes. . . . So to hell with the philosophy of the great men of the world" (to Suvorin, Dec. 17, 1890).

The older man could not comprehend why Chekhov did not advocate a particular moral point of view in his writing. Chekhov, on the other hand, had a different conception of the writer's role. He strove to be objective, to present people as they are, to present the world as it is. His medical training taught him to be a careful observer; his medical attitude made him leery of judging others. Chekhov presented his negative responses to Tolstoy's ideas in several of his mature stories, especially "The Duel" (1891), "An Artist's Story" (1896), and "My Life" (1896). Nonetheless, despite their differences, Chekhov revered the aged master.

Although Tolstoy focused on a morality of radical communalism, many other writers and intellectuals of the time spoke out against Russia's repressive social and political institutions. Much of this protest was disguised in various ways to satisfy the omnipresent state censors, but late-nineteenth-century Russians (like their twentieth-century counterparts) learned to speak and understand a subtle code of protest. The intellectuals addressed "big issues"—democracy, education, and social revolution. They wrote articles and organized meetings and gave speeches. Here again, Chekhov seemed to be on a different wavelength. He rarely engaged in theoretical discussion of these issues (at least publicly), and he did not advocate radical social change. Rather, as we have seen, he preferred a pragmatic, case-based approach. His goals were relatively limited, but achievable. Treat the sick patient. Document and publicize the abysmal condition of prisoners on Sakhalin Island. Contain the cholera epidemic. Provide financial assistance to keep farmers afloat during the famine. Raise money for a new school. It goes on and on but is always specific and personal.

In the long run Chekhov's objectivity and aversion to theory played a major role in the development of modern literature. Twentieth-century writers followed Chekhov in attempting to describe the world of human character and relationship objectively, and allowing that world to speak for itself. Contrary to the beliefs of critics who argued that Chekhov's work had no moral center, the moral dimension of Chekhov's writing is firmly rooted in the individual. The moral stories of Chekhov's world arise from the relationships among weak, vulnerable people who have difficulty communicating with one another. They represent grassroots morality, not a moral or social theory imposed from above. Similarly, Chekhov's doctors are individuals, not representatives. Yet in the aggregate they reveal the author's deep understanding of human nature as it applies to the complex and often overwhelming profession of medicine.

3.

Chekhov also drew from his medical experience in creating a multitude of physician characters. Doctors play significant roles in thirty or so of Chekhov's stories and in every one of his major plays, except *The Cherry Orchard*. In most cases they function in specific medical situations or are the principal protagonists. In other cases the doctor is an observer or subsidiary character. The author's sensibility as a medical insider gives special insight and poignancy to these characters. These doctors demonstrate a wide spectrum of behavior, personality, and character. Some are committed, some are lazy, and some suffer from burnout. Many are pompous, several are drunks, and very few are heroes. Chekhov knew too much about medicine to think that his doctors could actually heal many people, or make the world a better place. Thus, his medical men and women often appear impotent. Yet their impotence provides an arena in which a moral drama takes place. They define themselves as moral beings by the manner in which they respond to the overwhelming nature of their task.

Chekhov's doctors provide an especially interesting vantage point from which to view their author's project. For one thing, their world is Chekhov's world. At their best they convey the seamless fabric of tenderness (compassion) and steadiness (detachment) that lies at the heart of good medical practice. In fact, some of them demonstrate the same imaginative attention that Dr. Chekhov himself gave to his patients and to his characters. Dr. Pavel Archangelsky, who supervised Chekhov's first job as a physician, captured the author's ability to listen carefully when he later commented on the young doctor's performance: "he did everything with attention and a manifest love of what he was doing, especially toward the patients who passed through his hands. He listened quietly to them, never raising his voice however tired he was and even if the patient was talking about things quite irrelevant to his illness" (as quoted in John Coope, *Doctor Chekhov: A Study in Literature and Medicine* [Chale, Isle of Wight: Cross Publishing, 1997], 27).

At their best, Chekhov's doctors also demonstrate courage, altruism, and self-effacement. Dr. Dymov in "The Grasshopper" (1892) dies as a result of his work taking care of diphtheria patients, and Dr. Thompson, an almost Christ-like figure in "The Head Gardener's Story" (1894), is murdered. Dr. Kirilov in "Enemies" (1887) demonstrates extraordinary devotion to duty by leaving his distraught wife and the body of his son to make what appears to be an emergency house call.

Perhaps Chekhov's most textured and realistic portrait of a good physician appears in the late story called "A Doctor's Visit" (1898). Interestingly, the protagonist, Korolyov, is a young doctor substituting for his boss, the professor of medicine. During the course of the story he moves from being a sensitive and careful observer (with detached concern) who ascertains that his patient has no organic problem to making an imaginative leap that leads him to connect more deeply with his patient and her story. This imaginative connection allows him to relieve some of her suffering by reframing her illness. He is unable to solve the existential problems that press heavily on her, but his demonstration of solidarity leads her to trust him and develop a better understanding of her problems. Korolyov's transformation is not only characteristic of good medical practice, it is also emblematic of Chekhov's approach to literature—a "privileging" of the individual in which the moral dimension arises from the case itself, rather than the case being used to illustrate an aspect of morality.

From what we know of Korolyov, it is reasonable to believe that his empathy and openness may protect him from the emotional slings and arrows that might damage others in a medical career. Although he displays a similar sense of social injustice, unlike the highly theoretical Dr. Blagovo in "My Life" (1896), Korolyov looks like he might avoid the mistake of championing revolutionary theories in lieu of doing constructive work. Korolyov appears too well grounded in the particular and too interested in individual human narratives to become a theorist. Likewise, I suspect that Korolyov would be comfortable acknowledging and using the power of the doctor–patient relationship to promote his patients' welfare, as does his fictional colleague, Marfa Petrovna Petchonkin ("Malingerers," 1885). I can imagine this young doctor in middle age, having become a well-liked and respected local physician like Samoylenko in "The Duel" (1891), a man who empathizes with them, respects them, and attempts to mediate their conflicts.

Other physician characters present us with surprising contradictions. In "Excellent People" (1886) Vera suffers from what today we might call an "existential crisis." After surviving a suicide attempt she appears to have given up medicine completely but then all of a sudden reactivates herself and goes off to become a public-health worker in the provinces. Dr. Tsvyetkov ("The Doctor," 1886) displays admirable compassion as he keeps vigil over the dying child of an unmarried woman, but at the same time we learn that he may well be the child's father. The doctor is desperate for the boy's mother to tell him the "truth"; he wants to hear that someone else is the father so that he can regain his professional reserve and need not experience the anguish of attending his own son's death. Another doctor who loses his cool is Mikhail Ivanovitch ("The Princess," 1889), who is working part time at a monastery. He and his former employer, the princess, meet at the monastery, and as they talk she implores the mild-mannered doctor to tell her about her faults. He responds with a full-fledged diatribe—the woman is a vain and heartless hypocrite. But almost as soon as these words are out of his mouth, the doctor backs off, expresses his humility, and tries to make amends.

At the other end of the spectrum, many of Chekhov's doctors are insensitive, incompetent, or impaired. Klotchkov, the callous medical student in "Anyuta" (1886), and Mayer, one of the students in "A Nervous Breakdown" (1889), are youthful versions of this professional type. Perhaps a few more years of experience will help these young men to become more empathic and compassionate, but that seems doubtful. Take Mayer, for example. He can quote accurate statistics on the numbers of whores in London and Moscow, but he is unable to "see" (empathize with) the suffering of the living-and-breathing whores he actually encounters. Or consider Klotchkov, who conceives of his mistress as an object to be discarded at the drop of a hat. Shelestov in "Intrigues" (1883) and the public health doctor in "Darkness" (1887) are examples of self-centered physicians a little further along in their professional lives. The former is superficial and pompous; the latter is narrow-minded and detached. Neither presents the face of healing.

Chekhov's most complete imagining of the doctor as an insensitive, acquisitive social climber is found in "Ionitch" (1898). Startsev, when the reader first meets him, is a young physician setting up practice in a provincial town. He appears earnest and energetic, albeit a bit self-important. After surviving an unrequited infatuation with Ykaterina, the daughter of a wealthy townsman, Startsev gets down to the business of medicine. His practice prospers, and he branches out into the real estate business. He grows corpulent and wealthy:

> Probably because his throat is covered with rolls of fat, his voice has changed; it has become thin and sharp. His temper has changed, too; he has become ill humored and irritable. When he sees his patients, he is usually out of temper; he impatiently taps the floor with his stick, and shouts in his disagreeable voice: "Be so good as to confine yourself to answering my questions! Don't talk so much!"

"Ionitch" traces the progressive change that may occur in a medical practitioner who finds that medical affluence is more to his liking than the emotionally and physically difficult path of medical virtue. The story begins when Startsev is young and relatively "unformed." His abortive romance with Ykaterina results in a conscious decision to harden himself and turn away from the world of emotional commitments. To avoid getting hurt a second time, Startsev will simply never again become emotionally involved. He becomes detached to the point that he cannot "see" the suffering of others. Although "Ionitch" places this change in a romantic context, the outcome parallels that of "clinical distance" or "detached concern," in which the vulnerable doctor gradually comes to look on emotion as his enemy in the quest for objectivity in medical practice.

Some of Chekhov's most interesting doctors are those whose hearts are tortured by existential or spiritual conflict. At one level, this conflict might deserve a clinical description. Chekhov accurately depicted many of the symptoms of "burnout," the syndrome of depletion, detachment, depersonalization, denial, and depression that plagues some physicians. Emotional detachment from family and friends is a relatively early phase. Dr. Kirilov, who chooses to "go to the office" instead of mourning with his wife, may illustrate this condition. Dr. Ovchinnikov in "An Awkward Business" (1888) presents the more advanced symptom of depersonalization when he slugs his assistant because of frustration over the man's incompetence. Clearly, Ovchinnikov is overworked, the hospital resources are inadequate, and the doctor feels impotent. However, he responds by objectifying and dehumanizing his assistant, a response that threatens to compromise the work that he was trying to protect. Dr. Chebutykin in *The Three Sisters* (1900) illustrates the extreme end of the burnout spectrum, where the process has resulted in chemical dependency. Though still employed as a military physician, Chebutykin makes no claim to be a "real" doctor. In fact, he convincingly asserts that he has forgotten all he ever learned about medicine. All that remains of him is an alcoholic husk.

Ragin ("Ward No. 6," 1892) and Nikolai Stepanovich ("A Dreary Story," 1889) are complex characters in whom depression and burnout are superimposed on (or accentuate) their deep sense of having been failures in life. Chekhov's characters typically suffer from a lack of self-knowledge, wandering through their lives relying on one form of self-deception or another, and often causing pain and miscommunication in their wake. Ragin and Stepanovich fill that bill. When they were younger, they apparently meant well. They committed themselves to useful enterprises—Stepanovich to academic medicine and Ragin to a life of service in provincial medical practice. However, in the long run the center didn't hold and they failed. They never "found" themselves. Professor Stepanovich experiences this failure as a yearning for a unifying moral principle that would meld together the fragments of his life. Dr. Ragin experiences the failure as emotional numbness, an inability to feel. He yearns to experience suffering, because at least if he felt physical or emotional pain, he would be freed from the prison of dullness or numbness in which he dwells. Thus, the academic physician pines for cognitive salvation; the practitioner pines for emotional redemption. In both cases they remain wedded to themselves rather than to a concern for others, in whom salvation might actually be found.

Ragin and Stepanovich are physicians, of course, and they perhaps at one level illustrate the perils of clinical detachment taken too far, but their spiritual crisis is common to all of us—the search for meaning in our lives. This was a quest that Chekhov himself faced soberly, with a cold eye and a warm heart.

An anthology that included all of Chekhov's doctors would be cumbersome indeed, roughly the size of a medical textbook. I intended this collection to be considerably lighter (at least in weight), as well as more enjoyable to read than *Harrison's Textbook of Internal Medicine.* Many of the doctors had to be left out, but which were they? To a large extent, the nature of the texts dictated my exclusion criteria. First, I was unable to present doctors that appear in Chekhov's plays. This is unfortunate because physicians play major roles in four of Chekhov's five full-length dramas—Drs. Lvov in *Ivanov,* Dorn in *The Seagull,* Astrov in *Uncle Vanya,* and Chebutykin in *The Three Sisters.* However, it would be difficult to characterize any of these individuals without including the entire text. Even if I could identify a single scene that captured the "essence" of the character, the benefits of including that scene would likely be outweighed by the burdens. This collection is meant to be thoroughly readable and enjoyable, and I doubt whether a single scene or part of a scene from one or more of the plays, even if preceded by a summary of the story, would be attractive on its own merits. Likewise, I had to exclude the doctors portrayed in "The Duel" (Samoylenko) and "My Life" (Blagovo). To include one or both of these novellas would severely compromise the space available for their colleagues in shorter stories.

The inclusion criteria for the remaining pieces were far less quantitative. I wanted to include stories in which the doctor character played a major role and in which medicine itself makes more than a cameo appearance. The fact that Sobol in "The Wife" (1892) is a physician may represent a feature of his character that Chekhov wishes to communicate to the reader. Nonetheless, "The Wife" is neither Sobol's story, nor medicine's story. Likewise, the doctor makes a fine narrator in "The Lights" (1888), but the tale would do just as well if he were a young lawyer or landowner. I also wanted to avoid repetition, so I would not have included more than one of the three stories, "Perpetuum Mobile" (1884), "The Examining Magistrate" (1887), and "On Official Business" (1899), each of which depicts a magistrate and a physician on their way to an inquest. In the end I elected to use "The Examining Magistrate" in response to my final inclusion criterion—personal preference. I wanted to share with you the stories that I like most. I hope you enjoy them, too.

CHEKHOV'S DOCTORS

Intrigues

a. Election of new chairman of the Association.
b. Discussion of the October 2nd incident.
c. Synopsis of the activities of member Dr. M. H. von Bronn.
d. Routine matters concerning the Association.

Doctor Shelestov, the culprit in the October 2nd incident, is getting ready to go to the meeting. He has been standing for a long time in front of the mirror, trying to give his face a languid look. If he were to turn up at the meeting with a face that looked concerned, tense, red, or slightly pale, then his enemies would deduce that he was affected by their intrigues. If his face was cold, impassive, as if he had had a good night's sleep, the kind of face that people have who are untouched by the toils and strife of life, then all his enemies would secretly be overcome with respect and think:

> *His proud rebellious head doth rise higher*
> *Than the giddying heights of Napoleon's*
> *monument.*

Like a person who has little interest in intrigues and squabbles, he would arrive at the meeting later than all the others. He would enter the room quietly, languidly pass his hand through his hair, and without looking at a single person, take a seat at the very end of the table. Assuming the pose of the bored listener, he would suppress a yawn, pick up a newspaper, and start reading. Everyone would be talking, arguing, boiling over, calling each other to order—but he would remain silent, reading his newspaper. Then finally, as his name was repeated more and more often and the burning question turned whitehot, he would lift his bored, weary eyes to say to his colleagues, reluctantly:

"You are forcing me to speak . . . Gentleman, I have not prepared a speech, so please bear with me—my words cannot do this scandal justice. I shall begin *ab ovo*. At the last meeting some of our esteemed colleagues asserted that I do not conduct myself in an appropriate manner during medical consultations, and consequently they called me to account. Being of the opinion that I need not proffer justifications, and that the accusations are nothing but unscrupulous ploys, I asked that my name be removed from the membership roster of the Association, and subsequently resigned. Now, however, that a whole series of new accusations are being leveled against me, I find, to my great regret, that I am forced to offer an explanation after all. With your permission, I shall explain."

At this point, carelessly twirling a pencil or a chain, he would say that yes, in actual fact it was true that during consultations he had sometimes been known to raise his voice and attack colleagues, regardless of who was present. It was also true that once, during a consultation, in the presence of doctors and family members, he had asked the patient, "Who was the idiot who prescribed opium for you?" Rare was a consultation without incident . . . But why was this? The answer was simple! In these consultations he, Shelestov, was always saddled with colleagues whose knowledge left much to be desired. There were thirty-two doctors in town, most of whom knew less than a first-year medical student. One didn't have to look far for examples. Needless to say, *nomina sunt odiosa*—one does not wish to name names—but as they were among themselves at the meeting, and he did not want to appear a scandalmonger, names would be mentioned. For instance, everyone was aware that our esteemed colleague von Bronn pierced the esophagus of Madam Seryozhkina, the official's wife, when he inserted a probe.

At that point von Bronn would jump up, wring his hands, and cry out: "My dear colleague, you were the one who stabbed her, not I! I'll prove it!"

Shelestov would ignore him, and continue: "Furthermore, as everyone is aware, our esteemed colleague Zhila mistook the actress Semiramidina's floating kidney for an abscess and undertook a probing puncture. The immediate result was *exitus letalis*—lethal consequences! Our esteemed friend Besstrunko, instead of removing the nail from the big toe of a left foot, removed the healthy nail from the right foot. I am also pressed to recall the case in which our esteemed colleague Terkhayantz catheterized the soldier Ivanov's eustachian tubes with such vigor that both his eardrums exploded. I would also like to remind you that this very same colleague of ours, while extracting a tooth, dislocated the patient's lower jaw and wouldn't reset it until the patient agreed to pay him five rubles for the procedure. Our esteemed colleague Kuritsin, who is married to the pharmacist Grommet's niece, is running a racket with him. Everyone is also aware that the secretary of our Association, your young friend Skoropalitelni, is living with the wife of our highly valued and esteemed chairman, Gustav Gustavovitch Prechtel. You will notice that I have delicately moved from discussing lack of medical knowledge to unethical behavior. I have no choice! Ethics is our weak point, gentlemen, and so as not to appear a mere scandalmonger, I will call to your attention our esteemed colleague Puzirkov, who at Colonel Treshinskay's name-day party told everyone that it was not Skoropalitelni who was living with our chairman's wife, but I! The effrontery of Mr. Puzirkov, whom I myself caught last year with the wife of our esteemed colleague, Dr. Znobish! Speaking of Znobish—who is it that uses his position as a doctor and can't quite be trusted when treating ladies? Znobish! Who is it that married a merchant's daughter for her dowry? Znobish! And as for our highly esteemed chairman, he secretly dabbles in homeopathy and receives money from the Prussians for espionage! A Prussian spy—that is the *ultima ratio!*"

When doctors wish to appear clever and eloquent they use two Latin expressions: *nomina sunt odiosa* and *ultima ratio.* Shelestov would drop not only Latin words but French and German ones as well—whatever you want. He would steer everyone to clear waters, rip the masks off the intriguer's faces. The chairman would ring his bell till he was exhausted—esteemed colleagues would be flying up from their seats all over the place, yelling and waving their arms—colleagues of every denomination would fall over each other in a heap:

Zip-bang-wham-bang-wham-bang-wham!

Not batting an eyelash, Shelestov would continue: "And as for this Association, its current membership and organization, being what it is, it is inevitably headed for destruction. Its whole structure is based exclusively on intrigues. Intrigues, intrigues, intrigues! I, as one of the victims of a mass of demonic intrigues, consider myself bound to expound the following. . . ."

He would go on expounding, and his supporters would applaud and clasp their hands together in exultation. At this point, with an unimaginable uproar and appeals of thunder, the voting for the new chairman would commence. Von Bronn and his cohorts would heatedly support Prechtel, but the public and the ethical group of doctors would boo them and shout. "Down with Prechtel! We want Shelestov! Shelestov!"

Shelestov would consent, but on condition that Prechtel and von Bronn ask his forgiveness for the October 2nd incident. Again there would be an unimaginable clamor, and again the esteemed colleagues of the Jewish faith would fall over each other in a heap: "Zip-bang-wham!" Prechtel and von Bronn, seething with indignation, would end up resigning from the Association. Not that he would care!

Shelestov would end up as chairman. First he would clean out the Augean stables. Znobish—out! Terkhanayantz—out! The esteemed colleagues of the Jewish denomination—out! With his supporters he would see to it that by January not a single intriguer would be left in the Association. The first thing he would do would be to have the walls of the Association's clinic painted, and hang up a sign saying "Absolutely No Smoking." Then he would fire the medical attendant and his wife, and medicine would henceforth be ordered not from the Grumer pharmacy but from the Khryashchambzhitdkov pharmacy. All doctors would be forbidden to perform operations without his supervision, etc. And most important, he would have visiting cards printed, saying "Chairman of the Association of Doctors."

Thus Shelestov dreams as he stands at home in front of his mirror. But the clock strikes seven, reminding him that it is time to leave for the meeting. He shakes himself awake from his sweet thoughts and hurriedly tries to give his face a languid expression, but—alas! He tries to make his face languid and interesting, but it does not obey, and instead becomes sour and dull, like the face of a shivering mongrel puppy. He tries to make his face look firm, but it resists and expresses bewilderment, and it seems to him now that he does not look like a puppy but like a goose. He lowers his eyelids, narrows his eyes, puffs up his cheeks, knits his brow, but all to no avail . . . damn! . . . he cannot get the right expression. Obviously, the innate characteristics of that face are such that you couldn't do much with them. His forehead is narrow, his small eyes flit about nervously, like those of a cunning marketwoman; his lower jaw juts out somehow absurdly and stupidly; and his cheeks and hair give the impression that this "esteemed colleague" has just been kicked out of a billiard parlor.

Shelestov looks at his face, flies into a rage, and begins sensing that his face is plotting against him. He goes out into the hall, and as he is putting on his coat, his galoshes, and his hat, he feels that they are intriguing against him too.

"Cabbie, to the clinic!"

He hands the cabbie twenty kopecks, and the intriguing cabbie asks for twenty-five. He sits in the droshky going down the street; the cold wind beats him in the face, the wet snow flies into his eyes, the horse drags its feet. Everything is conspiring to intrigue against him. Intrigues, intrigues, intrigues!

Malingerers

Marfa Petrovna Petchonkin, the General's widow, who has been practicing for ten years as a homeopathic doctor, is seeing patients in her study on one of the Tuesdays in May. On the table before her lie a chest of homeopathic drugs, a book on homeopathy, and bills from a homeopathic chemist. On the wall the letters from some Petersburg homeopath, in Marfa Petrovna's opinion a very celebrated and great man, hang under glass in a gilt frame, and there also is a portrait of Father Aristark, to whom the lady owes her salvation—that is, the renunciation of pernicious allopathy and the knowledge of the truth. In the vestibule patients are sitting waiting, for the most part peasants. All but two or three of them are barefoot, as the lady has given orders that their ill-smelling boots are to be left in the yard.

Marfa Petrovna has already seen ten patients when she calls the eleventh: "Gavrila Gruzd!"

The door opens and instead of Gavrila Gruzd, Zamuhrishen, a neighboring landowner who has sunk into poverty, a little old man with sour eyes, and with a gentleman's cap under his arm, walks into the room. He puts down his stick in the corner, goes up to the lady, and without a word drops on one knee before her.

"What are you about, Kuzma Kuzmitch?" cries the lady in horror, flushing crimson. "For goodness sake!"

"While I live I will not rise," says Zamuhrishen, bending over her hand. "Let all the world see my homage on my knees, our guardian angel, benefactress of the human race! Let them! Before the good fairy who has given me life, guided me into the path of truth, and enlightened my skepticism I am ready not merely to kneel but to pass through fire, our miraculous healer, mother of the orphan and the widowed! I have recovered. I am a new man, enchantress!"

"I . . . I am very glad," mutters the lady, flushing with pleasure. "It's so pleasant to hear that. Sit down please! Why, you were so seriously ill that Tuesday."

"Yes indeed, how ill I was! It's awful to recall it," says Zamuhrishen, taking a seat. "I had rheumatism in every part and every organ. I have been in misery for eight years. I've had no rest from it . . . by day or by night, my benefactress. I have consulted doctors, and I went to professors at Kazan; I have tried all sorts of

5

mud-baths, and drunk waters, and goodness knows what I haven't tried! I have wasted all my substance on doctors, my beautiful lady. The doctors did me nothing but harm. They drove the disease inwards. Drive in, that they did, but to drive out was beyond their science. All they care about is their fees, the brigands; but as for the benefit of humanity—for that they don't care a straw. They prescribe some quackery, and you have to drink it. Assassins, that's the only word for them. If it hadn't been for you, our angel, I should have been in the grave by now! I went home from you that Tuesday, looked at the pilules that you gave me then, and wondered what good there could be in them. Was it possible that those little grains, scarcely visible, could cure my immense, long-standing disease? That's what I thought—unbeliever that I was!—and I smiled; but when I took the pilule it was instantaneous! It was as though I had not been ill, or as though it had been lifted off me. My wife looked at me with her eyes starting out of her head and couldn't believe it. 'Why, is it you, Kolya?' 'Yes, it is I,' I said. And we knelt down together before the icon, and fell to praying for our angel: 'Send her, O Lord, all that we are feeling!'"

Zamuhrishen wipes his eyes with his sleeve, gets up from his chair, and shows a disposition to drop on one knee again; but the lady checks him and makes him sit down.

"It's not me you must thank," she says, blushing with excitement and looking enthusiastically at the portrait of Father Aristark. "It's not my doing. I am only the obedient instrument . . . It's really a miracle. Rheumatism of eight years' standing by one pilule of scrofuloso!"

"Excuse me, you were so kind as to give me three pilules. One I took at dinner and the effect was instantaneous! Another in the evening, and the third next day; and since then not a touch! Not a twinge anywhere! And you know I thought I was dying, I had written to Moscow for my son to come! The Lord has given you wisdom, our lady of healing! Now I am walking, and feel as though I were in Paradise. The Tuesday I came to you I was hobbling, and now I am ready to run after a hare. . . . I could live for a hundred years. There's only one trouble, our lack of means. I'm well now, but what's the use of health if there's nothing to live on? Poverty weighs on me worse than illness. . . . For example, take this . . . It's the time to sow oats, and how is one to sow it if one has no seed? I ought to buy it, but the money . . . everyone knows how we are off for money."

"I will give you oats, Kuzma Kuzmitch. . . . Sit down, sit down. You have so delighted me; you have given me so much pleasure that it's not you but I that should say thank you!"

"You are our joy! That the Lord should create such goodness! Rejoice, Madam, looking at your good deeds! . . . While we sinners have no cause or rejoicing in ourselves. . . . We are paltry, poor-spirited, useless people . . . a mean lot. . . . We are only gentry in name, but in a material sense we are the same as peasants, only worse. . . . We live in stone houses, but it's a mere make-believe . . . for the roof leaks. And there is no money to buy wood to mend it with."

"I'll give you the wood, Kuzma Kuzmitch."

Zamuhrishen asks for and gets a cow too, a letter of recommendation for his daughter whom he wants to send to a boarding school, and . . . touched by the lady's liberality he whimpers with excess of feeling, twists his mouth, and feels in his pocket for his handkerchief.

Marfa Petrovna sees a red paper slip out of his pocket with his handkerchief and fall noiselessly to the floor.

"I shall never forget it to all eternity," he mutters, "and I shall make my children and my grandchildren remember it . . . from generation to generation. 'See, children,' I shall say, 'who, has saved me from the grave, who . . . '"

When she has seen her patient out, the lady looks for a minute at Father Aristark with eyes full of tears, then turns her caressing, reverent gaze on the drug chest, the books, the bills, the armchair in which the man she had saved from death has just been sitting, and her eyes fall on the paper just dropped by her patient. She picks up the paper, unfolds it, and sees in it three pilules—the very pilules she had given Zamuhrishen the previous Tuesday.

"They are the very ones," she thinks puzzled. "The paper is the same. . . . He hasn't even unwrapped them! What has he taken then? Strange. . . . Surely he wouldn't try to deceive me!"

And for the first time in her ten years of practice a doubt creeps into Marfa Petrovna's mind. . . . She summons the other patients, and while talking to them of their complaints notices what has hitherto slipped by her ears unnoticed. The patients, every one of them as though they were in a conspiracy, first belaud her for their miraculous cure, go into raptures over her medical skill, and abuse allopath doctors, then when she is flushed with excitement, begin holding forth on their needs. One asks for a bit of land to plough, another for wood, a third time for permission to shoot in her forests, and so on. She looks at the broad, benevolent countenance of Father Aristark who has revealed the truth to her, and a new truth begins gnawing at her heart. An evil oppressive truth.

The deceitfulness of man!

Excellent People

Once upon a time there lived in Moscow a man called Vladimir Semyonitch Liadovsky. He took his degree at the university in the faculty of law and had a post on the board of management of some railway; but if you had asked him what his work was, he would look candidly and openly at you with his large bright eyes through his gold pince-nez, and would answer in a soft, velvety, lisping baritone:

"My work is literature."

After completing his course at the university, Vladimir Semyonitch had had a paragraph of theatrical criticism accepted by a newspaper. From this paragraph he passed on to reviewing, and a year later he had advanced to writing a weekly article on literary matters for the same paper. But it does not follow from these facts that he was an amateur, that his literary work was of an ephemeral, haphazard character. Whenever I saw his neat spare figure, his high forehead and long mane of hair, when I listened to his speeches, it always seemed to me that his writing, quite apart from what and how he wrote, was something organically part of him, like the beating of his heart, and that his whole literary program must have been an integral part of his brain while he was a baby in his mother's womb. Even in his walk, his gestures, his manner of shaking of the ash from his cigarette, I could read this whole program from A to Z, with all its claptrap, dullness, and honorable sediments. He was a literary man all over when with an inspired face he laid a wreath on the coffin of some celebrity, or with a grave and solemn face collected signatures for some address; his passion for making the acquaintance of distinguished literary men, his faculty for finding talent even where it was absent, his perpetual enthusiasm, his pulse that went at one hundred and twenty a minute, his ignorance of life, the genuinely feminine flutter with which he threw himself into concerts and literary evenings for the benefit of destitute students, the way in which he gravitated towards the young— all this would have created for him the reputation of a writer even if he had not written his articles.

He was one of those writers to whom phrases like, "We are but few," or "What would life be without strife? Forward!" were pre-eminently becoming, though he never strove with any one and never did go forward. It did not even sound mawkish when he fell to discoursing of ideals. Every anniversary of the university, on St. Tatiana's Day, he got drunk, chanted *Gaudeamus* out of tune, and his beaming and perspiring countenance seemed to say: "See, I'm drunk; I'm keeping it up!" But even that suited him.

Vladimir Semyonitch had genuine faith in his literary vocation and his whole program. He had no doubts, and was evidently very well pleased with himself. Only one thing grieved him—the paper for which he worked had a limited circulation and was not very influential. But Vladimir Semyonitch believed that sooner or later he would succeed in getting on to a solid magazine where he would have scope and could display himself—and what little distress he felt on this score was pale beside the brilliance of his hopes.

Visiting this charming man, I made the acquaintance of his sister, Vera Semyonovna, a woman doctor. At first sight, what struck me about this woman was her look of exhaustion and extreme ill health. She was young, with a good figure and regular, rather large features, but in comparison with her agile, elegant, and talkative brother she seemed angular, listless, slovenly, and sullen. There was something strained, cold, apathetic in her movements, smiles, and words; she was not liked, and was thought proud and not very intelligent.

In reality, I fancy she was resting.

"My dear friend," her brother would often say to me, sighing and flinging back his hair in his picturesque literary way, "one must never judge by appearances! Look at this book: it has long ago been read. It is warped, tattered, and lies in the dust uncared for; but open it, and it will make you weep and turn pale. My sister is like that book. Lift the cover and peep into her soul, and you will be horror-stricken. Vera passed in some three months through experiences that would have been ample for a whole lifetime!"

Vladimir Semyonitch looked round him, took me by the sleeve, and began to whisper:

"You know, after taking her degree she married, for love, an architect. It's a complete tragedy! They had hardly been married a month when—whew—her husband died of typhus. But that was not all. She caught typhus from him, and when, on her recovery, she learnt that her Ivan was dead, she took a good dose of morphine. If it had not been for vigorous measures taken by her friends, my Vera would have been by now in Paradise. Tell me, isn't it a tragedy? And is not my sister like an *ingénue*, who has played already all the five acts of her life? The audience may stay for the farce, but the *ingénue* must go home to rest."

After three months of misery Vera Semyonovna had come to live with her brother. She was not fitted for the practice of medicine, which exhausted her and did not satisfy her; she did not give one the impression of knowing her subject, and I never once heard her say anything referring to her medical studies.

She gave up medicine, and, silent and unoccupied, as though she were a prisoner, spent the remainder of her youth in colorless apathy, with bowed head and hanging hands. The only thing to which she was not completely indifferent, and which brought some brightness into the twilight of her life, was the presence of her brother, whom she loved. She loved him himself and his program, she was full of reverence for his articles; and when she was asked what her brother was doing, she would answer in a subdued voice as though afraid of waking or distracting him: "He is writing." Usually when he was at his work she used to sit beside him, her eyes fixed on his writing hand. She used at such moments to look like a sick animal warming itself in the sun.

One winter evening Vladimir Semyonitch was sitting at his table writing a critical article for his newspaper: Vera Semyonovna was sitting beside him, staring as usual at his writing hand. The critic wrote rapidly, without erasures or corrections. The pen scratched and squeaked. On the table near the writing hand there lay open a freshly cut volume of a thick magazine, containing a story of peasant life, signed with two initials. Vladimir Semyonitch was enthusiastic; he thought the author was admirable in his handling of the subject, suggested Turgenev in his descriptions of nature, was truthful, and had an excellent knowledge of the life of the peasantry. The critic himself knew nothing of peasant life except from books and hearsay, but his feelings and his inner convictions forced him to believe the story. He foretold a brilliant future for the author, assured him he should await the conclusion of the story with great impatience, and so on.

"Fine story!" he said, flinging himself back in his chair and closing his eyes with pleasure. "The tone is extremely good."

Vera Semyonovna looked at him, yawned aloud, and suddenly asked an unexpected question. In the evening she had a habit of yawning nervously and asking short, abrupt questions, not always relevant.

"Volodya," she asked, "what is the meaning of non-resistance to evil?"

"Non-resistance to evil!" repeated her brother, opening his eyes.

"Yes. What do you understand by it?"

"You see, my dear, imagine that thieves or brigands attack you, and you, instead of . . ."

"No, give me a logical definition."

"A logical definition? Um! Well." Vladimir Semyonitch pondered. "Non-resistance to evil means an attitude of non-interference with regard to all that in the sphere of mortality is called evil."

Saying this, Vladimir Semyonitch bent over the table and took up a novel. This novel, written by a woman, dealt with the painfulness of the irregular position of a society lady who was living under the same roof with her lover and her illegitimate child. Vladimir Semyonitch was pleased with the excellent tendency of the story, the plot and the presentation of it. Making a brief summary of the novel, he selected the best passages and added to them in his account: "How true to reality, how living, how picturesque! The author is not merely an artist; he is also a subtle psychologist who can see into the hearts of his characters. Take, for example, this vivid description of the emotions of the heroine on meeting her husband," and so on.

"Volodya," Vera Semyonovna interrupted his critical effusions, "I've been haunted by a strange idea since yesterday. I keep wondering where we should all be if human life were ordered on the basis of non-resistance to evil?"

"In all probability, nowhere. Non-resistance to evil would give the full rein to the criminal will, and, to say nothing of civilization, this would leave not one stone standing upon another anywhere on earth."

"What would be left?"

"Bashi-Bazouke and brothels. In my next article I'll talk about that perhaps. Thank you for reminding me."

And a week later my friend kept his promise. That was just at the period—in the eighties—when people were beginning to talk and write of non-resistance, of the right to judge, to punish, to make war; when some people in our set were beginning to do without servants, to retire into the country, to work on the land, and to renounce animal food and carnal love.

After reading her brother's article, Vera Semyonovna pondered and hardly perceptibly shrugged her shoulders.

"Very nice!" she said. "But still there's a great deal I don't understand. For instance, in Leskov's story 'Belonging to the Cathedral' there is a queer gardener who sows for the benefit of all—for customers, for beggars, and any who care to steal. Did he behave sensibly?"

From his sister's tone and expression Vladimir Semyonitch saw that she did not like this article, and, almost for the first time in his life, his vanity as an author sustained a shock. With a shade of irritation he answered:

"Theft is immoral. To sow for thieves is to recognize the right of thieves to existence. What would you think if I were to establish a newspaper and, dividing it into sections, provide for blackmailing as well as for liberal ideas? Following the example of the gardener, I ought, logically, to provide a section for blackmailers, the intellectual scoundrels? Yes."

Vera Semyonovna made no answer. She got up from the table, moved languidly to the sofa and lay down.

"I don't know, I know nothing about it," she said musingly. "You are probably right, but it seems to me, I feel somehow, that there's something false in our resistance to evil, as though there were something concealed or unsaid. God knows, perhaps our methods of resisting evil belong to the category of prejudices which have become so deeply rooted in us, that we are incapable of parting with them, and therefore cannot form a correct judgment of them."

"How do you mean?"

"I don't know how to explain to you. Perhaps man is mistaken in thinking that he is obliged to resist evil and has a right to do so, just as he is mistaken in thinking, for instance, that the heart looks like an ace of hearts. It is very possible in resisting evil we ought not to use force, but to use what is the very opposite of force—if you, for instance, don't want this picture stolen from you, you ought to give it away rather than lock it up."

"That's clever, very clever! If I want to marry a rich, vulgar woman, she ought to prevent me from such a shabby action by hastening to make me an offer herself!"

The brother and sister talked till midnight without understanding each other. If any outsider had overheard them he would hardly have been able to make out what either of them was driving at.

They usually spent the evening at home. There were no friends' houses to which they could go, and they felt no need for friends; they only went to the theatre when there was a new play—such was the custom in literary circles—they did not go to concerts, for they did not care for music.

"You may think what you like," Vera Semyonovna began again the next day, "but for me the question is to a great extent settled. I am firmly convinced that I have no grounds for resisting evil directed against me personally. If they want to kill me, let them. My defending myself will not make the murderer better. All I have now to decide is the second half of the question: how I ought to behave to evil directed against my neighbors?"

"Vera, mind you don't become rabid!" said Vladimir Semyonitch, laughing. "I see non-resistance is becoming your *idée fixe!*"

He wanted to turn off these tedious conversations with a jest, but somehow it was beyond a jest; his smile was artificial and sour. His sister gave up sitting beside his table and gazing reverently at his writing hand, and he felt every evening that behind him on the sofa lay a person who did not agree with him. And his back grew stiff and numb, and there was a chill in his soul. An author's vanity is vindictive, implacable, incapable of forgiveness, and his sister was the first and only person who had laid bare and disturbed that uneasy feeling, which is like a big box of crockery, easy to unpack but impossible to pack up again as it was before.

Weeks and months passed by, and his sister clung to her ideas, and did not sit down by the table. One spring evening Vladimir Semyonitch was sitting at his table writing an article. He was reviewing a novel which described how a village schoolmistress refused the man whom she loved and who loved her, a man both wealthy and intellectual, simply because marriage made her work as a schoolmistress impossible. Vera Semyonovna lay on the sofa and brooded.

"My God, how slow it is!" she said, stretching. "How insipid and empty life is! I don't know what to do with myself, and you are wasting your best years in goodness knows what. Like some alchemist, you are rummaging in old rubbish that nobody wants. My God!"

Vladimir Semyonitch dropped his pen and slowly looked round at his sister.

"It's depressing to look at you!" said his sister. "Wagner in 'Faust' dug up worms, but he was looking for treasure, anyway, and you are looking for worms for the sake of the worms."

"That's vague!"

"Yes, Volodya; all these days I've been thinking, I've been thinking painfully for a long time, and I have come to the conclusion that you are hopelessly reactionary and conventional. Come, ask yourself what is the object of your zealous, conscientious work? Tell me, what is it? Why, everything has long ago been extracted that can be extracted from that rubbish in which you are always rummaging. You may pound water in a mortar and analyze it as long as you like, you'll make nothing more of it than the chemists have made already."

"Indeed!" drawled Vladimir Semyonitch, getting up. "Yes, all this is old rubbish because these ideas are eternal; but what do you consider new, then?"

"You undertake to work in the domain of thought; it is for you to think of something new. It's not for me to teach you."

"Me—an alchemist!!" the critic cried in wonder and indignation, screwing up his eyes ironically. "Art, progress—all that is alchemy?"

"You see, Volodya, it seems to me that if all you thinking people had set yourselves to solving great problems, all these little questions that you fuss about now would solve themselves by the way. If you go up in a balloon to see a town, you will incidentally, without any effort, see the fields and the villages and the rivers as well. When stearine is manufactured, you get glycerin as a by-product. It seems to me that contemporary thought has settled on one spot and stuck to it. It is prejudiced, apathetic, timid, afraid to take a wide titanic flight, just as you and I are afraid to climb on a high mountain; it is conservative."

Such conversations could not but leave traces. The relations of the brother and sister grew more and more strained every day. The brother became unable to work in his sister's presence, and grew irritable when he knew his sister was lying on the sofa, looking at his back; while the sister frowned nervously and stretched when, trying to bring back the past, he attempted to share his enthusiasms with her. Every evening she complained of being bored, and talked about independence of mind and those who are in the rut of tradition. Carried away by her new ideas, Vera Semyonovna proved that the work that her brother was so engrossed in was conventional, that it was a vain effort of conservative minds to preserve what had already served its turn and was vanishing from the scene of action. She made no end of comparisons. She compared her brother at one time to an alchemist, then to a musty old Believer who would sooner die than listen to reason. By degrees there was a perceptible change in her manner of life, too. She was capable of lying on the sofa all day long doing nothing but think, while her face wore a cold, dry expression such as one sees in one-sided people of strong faith. She began to refuse the attentions of the servants, swept and tidied her own room, cleaned her own boots and brushed her own clothes. Her brother could not help looking with irritation and even hatred at her cold face when she went about her menial work. In that work, which was always performed with a certain solemnity, he saw something strained and false, he saw something both pharisa- ical and affected. And knowing he could not touch her by persuasion, he carped at her and teased her like a schoolboy.

"You won't resist evil, but you resist my having servants!" he taunted her. "If servants are an evil, why do you oppose it? That's inconsistent!"

He suffered, was indignant and even ashamed. He felt ashamed when his sis- ter began doing odd things before strangers.

"It's awful, my dear fellow," he said to me in private, waving his hands in de- spair. "It seems that our *ingénue* has remained to play a part in the farce, too. She's become morbid to the marrow of her bones! I've washed my hands of her, let her think as she likes; but why does she talk, why does she excite me? She ought to think what it means for me to listen to her. What I feel when in my presence she has the effrontery to support her errors by blasphemously quoting the teaching of Christ! It chokes me! It makes me hot all over to hear my sister propounding her doctrines and trying to distort the Gospel to suit her, when she purposely refrains from mentioning how the moneychangers were driven out of the Temple. That's, my dear fellow, what comes of being half educated, underdeveloped! That's what comes of medical studies which provide no general culture!"

One day on coming home from the office, Vladimir Semyonitch found his sister crying. She was sitting on the sofa with her head bowed, wringing her hands, and tears were flowing freely down her cheeks. The critic's good heart throbbed with pain. Tears fell from his eyes, too, and he longed to pet his sister, to forgive her, to beg her forgiveness, and to live as they used to before. . . . He knelt down and kissed her head, her hands, her shoulders. She smiled, smiled bitterly, unaccount- ably, while he with a cry of joy jumped up, seized the magazine from the table and said warmly:

"Hurrah! We'll live as we used to, Verotchka! With God's blessing! And I've such a surprise for you here! Instead of celebrating the occasion with champagne, let us read it together! A splendid, wonderful thing."

"Oh, no, no!" cried Vera Semyonovna, pushing away the book in alarm. "I've read it already! I don't want it, I don't want it!"

"When did you read it?"

"A year . . . two years ago. . . . I read it long ago, and I know it, I know it!"

"Hmm . . . You're a fanatic!" her brother said coldly, flinging the magazine on to the table.

"No, you are a fanatic, not I! You!" And Vera Semyonovna dissolved into tears again. Her brother stood before her, looked at her quivering shoulders, and thought. He thought, not of the agonies of loneliness endured by any one who begins to think in a new way of their own, not of the inevitable sufferings of a genuine spiritual revolution, but of the outrage of his program, the outrage to his author's vanity.

From this time he treated his sister coldly, with careless irony, and he endured her presence in the room as one endures the presence of old women that are dependent on one. For her part, she left off disputing with him and met all his arguments, jeers, and attacks with a condescending silence, which irritated him more than ever.

One summer morning Vera Semyonovna, dressed for traveling with a satchel over shoulder, went in to her brother and coldly kissed him on the forehead.

"Where are you going?" he asked with surprise.

"To the province of N. to do vaccination work." Her brother went out into the street with her.

"So that's what you've decided upon, you queer girl," he muttered. "Don't you want some money?"

"No, thank you. Good-bye."

The sister shook her brother's hand and set off.

"Why don't you have a cab?" cried Vladimir Semyonitch.

She did not answer. Her brother gazed after her, watched her rusty-looking waterproof, the swaying of her figure as she slouched along, forced himself to sigh, but did not succeed in rousing a feeling of regret. His sister had become a stranger to him. And he was a stranger to her. Anyway, she did not once look round.

Going back to his room, Vladimir Semyonitch at once sat down to the table and began to work at his article.

I never saw Vera Semyonovna again. Where she is now I do not know. And Vladimir Semyonitch went on writing articles, laying wreaths on coffins, singing *Gaudeamus,* busying himself over the Mutual Aid Society of Moscow Journalists.

He fell ill with inflammation of the lungs; he was ill in bed for three months—at first at home, and afterwards in the Golitsyn Hospital. An abscess developed on his knee. People said he ought to be sent to the Crimea, and began getting up a collection for him. But he did not go to the Crimea—he died. We buried him in the Vagankovsky Cemetery, on the left side, where artists and literary men are buried. One day we writers were sitting in the Tatars' Restaurant. I mentioned that

I had lately been in the Vagankovsky Cemetery and had seen Vladimir Semyon-itch's grave there. It was utterly neglected and almost indistinguishable from the rest of the ground, the cross had fallen; it was necessary to collect a few rubles to put it in order.

But they listened to what I said unconcernedly, made no answer, and I could not collect a farthing. No one remembered Vladimir Semyonitch. He was utterly forgotten.

Anyuta

In the cheapest room of a big block of furnished apartments Stepan Klotchkov, a medical student in his third year, was walking to and fro, zealously conning his anatomy. His mouth was dry and his forehead perspiring from the unceasing effort to learn it by heart.

In the window, covered by patterns of frost, sat on a stool the girl who shared his room—Anyuta, a thin little brunette of five-and-twenty, very pale with mild gray eyes. Sitting with bent back she was busy embroidering with red thread the collar of a man's shirt. She was working against time. The clock in the passage struck two drowsily, yet the little room had not been put to rights for the morning. Crumpled bed-clothes, pillows thrown about, books, clothes, a big filthy slop pail filled with soapsuds in which cigarette ends were swimming, and the litter on the floor—all seemed as though purposely jumbled together in one confusion.

"The right lung consists of three parts. . . ." Klotchkov repeated. "Boundaries! Upper part on anterior wall of thorax reaches the fourth or fifth rib, on the lateral surface, the fourth rib behind to the *spina scapulae. . . .*"

Klotchkov raised his eyes to the ceiling, striving to visualize what he had just read. Unable to form a clear picture of it, he began feeling his upper ribs through his waistcoat.

"These ribs are like the keys of a piano," he said. "One must familiarize oneself with them somehow, if one is not to get muddled over them. One must study them in the skeleton and the living body. I say, Anyuta, let me pick them out."

Anyuta put down her sewing, took off her blouse, and straightened herself up. Klotchkov sat down facing her, frowned, and began counting her ribs.

"H'm! . . . One can't feel the first rib; it's behind the shoulder blade. . . . This must be the second rib. . . . Yes . . . this is the third . . . this is the fourth. . . . H'm! . . . Yes. . . . Why are you wriggling?"

"Your fingers are cold!"

"Come, come . . . it won't kill you. Don't twist about. That must be the third rib, then . . . this is the fourth . . . You look such a skinny thing, and yet one can hardly feel your ribs. That's the second . . . that's the third. . . . Oh, this is muddling, and one can't see it clearly . . . I must draw it. . . . Where's my crayon?"

Klotchkov took his crayon and drew on Anyuta's chest several parallel lines corresponding with the ribs.

"First-rate. That's all straightforward. Well, now I can sound you, stand up!"

Anyuta stood up and raised her chin. Klotchkov began sounding her, and was so absorbed in this occupation that he did not notice how Anyuta's lips, nose, and fingers turned blue with cold. Anyuta shivered, and was afraid the student, noticing it, would leave off drawing and sounding her, and then, perhaps, might fail in his exam.

"Now it's all clear," said Klotchkov when he had finished. "You sit like that and don't rub off the crayon, and meanwhile I'll learn up a little more."

And the student again began walking to and fro, repeating to himself. Anyuta, with black stripes across her chest, looking as though she had been tattooed, sat thinking, huddled up and shivering with cold. She said very little as a rule; she was always silent, thinking and thinking.

In the six or seven years of her wanderings from one furnished room to another, she had known five students like Klotchkov. Now they had all finished their studies, had gone out into the world, and, of course, like respectable people, had long ago forgotten her. One of them was living in Paris, two were doctors, the fourth was an artist, and the fifth was said to be already a professor. Klotchkov was the sixth. Soon he, too, would finish his studies and go out into the world. There was a fine future before him, no doubt, and Klotchkov probably would become a great man, but the present was anything but bright; Klotchkov had no tobacco and no tea, and there were only four lumps of sugar left. She must make haste and finish her embroidery, take it to the woman who had ordered it, and with the quarter ruble she would get for it, buy tea and tobacco.

"Can I come in?" asked a voice at the door.

Anyuta quickly threw a woolen shawl over her shoulders. Fetisov the artist walked in.

"I have come to ask you a favor," he began, addressing Klotchkov and glaring like a wild beast from under the long locks that hung over his brow. "Do me a favor; lend me your young lady just for a couple of hours! I'm painting a picture, you see, and I can't get on without a model."

"Oh, with pleasure," Klotchkov agreed. "Go along, Anyuta."

"The things I've had to put up with there," Anyuta murmured softly.

"Rubbish! The man's is asking you for the sake of art, and not for any sort of nonsense. Why not help him if you can?"

Anyuta began dressing.

"And what are you painting?" asked Klotchkov.

"Psyche; it's a fine subject. But it won't go, somehow. I have to keep painting from different models. Yesterday I was painting one with blue legs. 'Why are your legs blue?' I asked her. 'It's my stockings stained them,' she said. And you're still grinding! Lucky fellow! You have patience."

"Medicine's a job one can't get on with without grinding."

"H'm! . . . Excuse me, Klotchkov, but you do live like a pig! It's awful the way you live!"

"How do you mean? I can't help it . . . I only get twelve rubles a month from my father, and it's hard to live decently on that."

"Yes . . . yes . . ." said the artist, frowning with an air of disgust, "but, still, you might live better. . . . An educated man is in duty bound to have taste, isn't he? And goodness knows what it's like here! The bed not made, the slops, the dirt, yesterday's porridge in the plates. Tfoo!"

"That's true," said the student in confusion, "but Anyuta has had no time to-day to tidy up; she's been busy all the while."

When Anyuta and the artist had gone out, Klotchkov lay down on the sofa and began learning, lying down; then he accidentally dropped asleep, and wak-ing up an hour later, propped his head on his fists and sank into gloomy reflection. He recalled the artist's words that an educated man was in duty bound to have taste, and his surroundings actually struck him now as loathsome and revolting. He saw, as it were in his mind's eye, his own future; when he would see his pa-tients in his consulting-room, drink tea in a large dining-room in the company of his wife, a real lady. And now that slop pail in which the cigarette ends were swimming looked incredibly disgusting. Anyuta, too, rose before his imagina-tion—a plain, slovenly, pitiful figure—and he made up his mind to part with her at once, at all costs.

When, on coming back from the artist's, she took off her coat, he got up and said to her seriously:

"Look here, my good girl . . . sit down and listen. We must part! The fact is, I don't want to live with you any longer."

Anyuta had come back from the artist's worn out and exhausted. Standing so long as a model had made her face look thin and sunken, and her chin sharper than ever. She said nothing in answer to the student's words, only her lips began to tremble.

"You know we should have to part sooner or later, anyway," said the student. "You're a nice, good girl, and not a fool; you'll understand. . . ."

Anyuta put on her coat again, in silence wrapped up her embroidery in paper, gathered together her needles and thread: she found the screw of paper with the four lumps of sugar in the window, and laid it on the table by the books.

"That's . . . your sugar," she said softly, and turned away to conceal her tears.

"Why are you crying?" asked Klotchkov.

He walked about the room in confusion, and said:

"You are a strange girl, really . . . Why, you know we shall have to part. We can't stay together for ever."

She had gathered together all her belongings, and turned to say good-bye to him, and he felt sorry for her.

"Shall I let her stay on here another week?" he thought. "She really may as well stay, and I'll tell her to go in a week;" and vexed at his own weakness, he shouted to her roughly:

"Come, why are you standing there? If you are going, go; and if you don't want to, take off your coat and stay! You can stay!"

Anyuta took off her coat, silently, stealthily, then blew her nose also stealthily, sighed, and noiselessly returned to her invariable position on her stool by the window.

The student drew his textbook to him and began again pacing from corner to corner. "The right lung consists of three parts," he repeated; "the upper part, on anterior wall of thorax, reaches the fourth or fifth rib. . . ."

In the passage some one shouted at the top of his voice: "Grigory! The samovar!"

The Doctor

It was still in the drawing-room, so still that a house-fly that had flown in from outside could be distinctly heard brushing against the ceiling. Olga Ivanovna, the lady of the villa, was standing by the window, looking out at the flower-beds and thinking. Dr. Tsvyetkov, who was her doctor as well as an old friend, and had been sent for to treat her son Misha, was sitting in an easy chair and swinging his hat, which he held in both hands, and he too was thinking. Except them, there was not a soul in the drawing-room or in the adjoining rooms. The sun had set, and the shades of evening began settling in the corners under the furniture and on the cornices.

The silence was broken by Olga Ivanovna.

"No misfortune more terrible can be imagined," she said, without turning from the window. "You know that life has no value for me whatever apart from the boy."

"Yes, I know that," said the doctor.

"No value whatever," said Olga Ivanovna, and her voice quivered. "He is everything to me. He is my joy, my happiness, my wealth. And if, as you say, I cease to be a mother, if he . . . dies, there will be nothing left of me but a shadow. I cannot survive it."

Wringing her hands, Olga Ivanovna walked from one window to the other and went on:

"When he was born, I wanted to send him away to the Foundling Hospital, you remember that, but, my God, how can that time be compared with now? Then I was vulgar, stupid feather-headed, but now I am a mother, do you understand? I am a mother, and that's all I care to know. Between the present and the past there is an impassable gulf."

Silence followed again. The doctor shifted his seat from the chair to the sofa and impatiently playing with his hat, kept his eyes fixed upon Olga Ivanovna. From his face it could be seen that he wanted to speak, and was waiting for a fitting moment.

"You are silent, but still I do not give up hope," said the lady, turning round.

"Why are you silent?"

"I should be as glad of any hope as you, Olga, but there is none," Tsvyetkov answered, "We must look the hideous truth in the face. The boy has a tumor on the brain, and we must try to prepare ourselves for his death, for such cases never recover."

"Nikolay, are you certain you are not mistaken?"

"Such questions lead to nothing. I am ready to answer as many as you like, but it will make it no better for us."

Olga Ivanovna pressed her face into the window curtains, and began weeping bitterly. The doctor got up and walked several times up and down the drawing-room, then went to the weeping woman, and lightly touched her arm. Judging from his uncertain movements, from the expression of his gloomy face, which looked dark in the dusk of the evening, he wanted to say something.

"Listen, Olga," he began. "Spare me a minute's attention; there is something I must ask you. You can't attend to me now, though. I'll come later, afterwards...." He sat down again, and sank into thought. The bitter, imploring weeping, like the weeping of a little girl, continued. Without waiting for it to end, Tsvyetkov heaved a sigh and walked out of the drawing room. He went into the nursery to Misha. The boy was lying on his back as before, staring at one point as though he were listening. The doctor sat down on his bed and felt his pulse.

"Misha, does your head ache?" he asked.

Misha answered, not at once: "Yes. I keep dreaming."

"What do you dream?"

"All sorts of things. . . ."

The doctor, who did not know how to talk with weeping women or with children, stroked his burning head, and muttered:

"Never mind, poor boy, never mind . . . One can't go through life without illness. . . . Misha, who am I—do you know me?"

Misha did not answer.

"Does your head ache very badly?"

"Ve-ery. I keep dreaming."

After examining him and putting a few questions to the maid who was looking after the sick child, the doctor went slowly back to the drawing-room. There it was by now dark, and Olga Ivanovna, standing by the window, looked like a silhouette.

"Shall I light up?" asked Tsvyetkov.

No answer followed. The house-fly was still brushing against the ceiling. Not a sound floated in from outside as though the whole world, like the doctor, were thinking, and could not bring itself to speak. Olga Ivanovna was not weeping now, but as before, staring at the flower-bed in profound silence. When Tsvyetkov went up to her, and through the twilight glanced at her pale face, exhausted with grief, her expression was such as he had seen before during her attacks of acute, stupefying, sick headache.

"Nikolay Trofimitch!" she addressed him, "and what do you think about a consultation?"

"Very good; I'll arrange it tomorrow."

From the doctor's tone it could be easily seen that he put little faith in the benefit of a consultation. Olga Ivanovna would have asked him something else, but her sobs prevented her. Again she pressed her face into the window curtain. At that moment, the strains of a band playing at the club floated in distinctly. They could hear not only the wind instruments, but even the violins and the flutes.

"If he is in pain, why is he silent?" asked Olga Ivanovna. "All day long, not a sound, he never complains, and never cries. I know God will take the poor boy from us because we have not known how to prize him. Such a treasure!"

The band finished the march, and a minute later began playing a lively waltz for the opening of the ball.

"Good God, can nothing really be done?" moaned Olga Ivanovna. "Nikolay, you are a doctor and ought to know what to do! You must understand that I can't bear the loss of him! I can't survive it."

The doctor, who did not know how to talk to weeping women, heaved a sigh, and paced slowly about the drawing-room. There followed a succession of oppressive pauses interspersed with weeping and the questions, which lead to nothing. The band had already played a quadrille, a polka, and another quadrille. It got quite dark. In the adjoining room, the maid lighted the lamp; and all the while the doctor kept his hat in his hands, and seemed trying to say something. Several times Olga Ivanovna went off to her son, sat by him for half an hour, and came back again into the drawing-room; she was continually breaking into tears and lamentations. The time dragged agonizingly, and it seemed as though the evening had no end.

At midnight, when the band had played the cotillion and ceased altogether, the doctor got ready to go.

"I will come again tomorrow," he said, pressing the mother's cold hand. "You go to bed."

After putting on his greatcoat in the passage and picking up his walking-stick, he stopped, thought a minute, and went back into the drawing-room.

"I'll come tomorrow, Olga," he repeated in a quivering voice. "Do you hear?"

She did not answer, and it seemed as though grief had robbed her of all power of speech. In his greatcoat and with his stick still in his hand, the doctor sat down beside her, and began in a soft, tender half whisper, which was utterly out of keeping with his heavy, dignified figure:

"Olga! For the sake of your sorrow which I share.... Now, when falsehood is criminal, I beseech you to tell me the truth. You have always declared that the boy is my son. Is that the truth?"

Olga Ivanovna was silent.

"You have been the one attachment in my life," the doctor went on, "and you cannot imagine how deeply my feeling is wounded by falsehood.... Come, I entreat you, Olga, for once in your life, tell me the truth.... At these moments one cannot lie. Tell me that Misha is not my son. I am waiting."

"He is."

Olga Ivanovna's face could not be seen, but in her voice the doctor could hear hesitation.

He sighed.

"Even at such moments you can bring yourself to tell a lie," he said in his ordinary voice. "There is nothing sacred to you! Do listen, do understand me.... You have been the one and only attachment in my life. Yes, you were depraved, vulgar, but I have loved no one else but you in my life. That trivial love, now that I am growing old, is the one solitary bright spot in my memories. Why do you darken it with deception? What is it for?"

"I don't understand you."

"Oh my God!" cried Tsvyetkov. "You are lying, you understand very well!" he cried more loudly, and he began pacing about the drawing room, angrily waving his stick. "Or have you forgotten? Then I will remind you! A father's rights to the boy are equally shared with me by Petrov and Kurovsky the lawyer, who still make you an allowance for their son's education, just as I do! Yes, indeed! I know all that quite well! I forgive your lying in the past, what does it matter? But now when you have grown older, at this moment when the boy is dying, your lying stifles me! How sorry I am that I cannot speak, how sorry I am!"

The doctor unbuttoned his overcoat, and still pacing about, said:

"Wretched woman! Even such moments have no effect on her! Even now she lies as freely as nine years ago in the Hermitage Restaurant! She is afraid if she tells me the truth I shall leave off giving her money, she thinks that if she did not lie I should not love the boy! You are lying! It's contemptible!"

The doctor rapped the floor with his stick, and cried:

"It's loathsome. Warped, corrupted creature! I must despise you, and I ought to be ashamed of my feeling. Yes! Your lying has stuck in my throat these nine years, I have endured it, but now it's too much—too much."

From the dark corner where Olga Ivanovna was sitting there came the sound of weeping. The doctor ceased speaking and cleared his throat. A silence followed. The doctor slowly buttoned up his overcoat, and began looking for his hat which he had dropped as he walked about.

"I lost my temper," he muttered, bending down to the floor. "I quite lost sight of the fact that you cannot attend to me now . . . God knows what I have said. . . . Don't take any notice of it, Olga."

He found his hat and went towards the dark corner.

"I have wounded you," he said in a soft, tender half-whisper, "but once more I entreat you, tell me the truth; there should not be lying between us. . . . I blurted it out, and now you know that Petrov and Kurovsky are no secret to me. So now it is easy for you to tell me the truth."

Olga Ivanovna thought a moment, and with perceptible hesitation, said:

"Nikolay, I am not lying—Misha is your child."

"My God," moaned the doctor, "then I will tell you something more: I have kept your letter to Petrov in which you call him Misha's father! Olga, I know the truth, but I want to hear it from you! Do you hear?"

Olga Ivanovna made no reply, but went on weeping. After waiting for an answer the doctor shrugged his shoulders and went out.

"I will come tomorrow," he called from the passage.

All the way home, as he sat in his carriage, he was shrugging his shoulders and muttering:

"What a pity that I don't know how to speak! I haven't the gift of persuading and convincing. It's evident she does not understand me since she lies! It's evident! How can I make her see? How?"

Darkness

A young peasant, with white eyebrows and eyelashes and broad cheekbones, in a torn sheepskin and big black felt overboots, waited till the Zemstvo doctor had finished seeing his patients and came out to go home from the hospital; then he went up to him, diffidently.

"Please, your honor," he said.

"What do you want?"

The young man passed the palm of his hand up and over his nose, looked at the sky, and then answered:

"Please, your honor. . . . You've got my brother Vaska the blacksmith from Varvarino in the convict ward here, your honor . . ."

"Yes, what then?"

"I am Vaska's brother, you see. . . . Father has the two of us: him, Vaska, and me, Kirila; besides us there are three sisters, and Vaska's a married man with a little one. . . . There are a lot of us and no one to work. . . . In the smithy it's nearly two years now since the forge has been heated. I am at the cotton factory, I can't do smith's work, and how can father work? Let alone work, he can't eat properly, he can't lift the spoon to his mouth."

"What do you want from me?"

"Be merciful! Let Vaska go!"

The doctor looked wonderingly at Kirila, and without saying a word walked on. The young peasant ran on in front and flung himself in a heap at his feet.

"Doctor, kind gentleman!" he besought him, blinking and again passing his open hand over his nose. "Show heavenly mercy; let Vaska go home! We shall remember you in our prayers forever! Your honor, let him go! They are all starving! Mother's wailing day in, day out, Vaska's wife's wailing . . . it's worse than death! I don't care to look upon the light of day. Be merciful; let him go, kind gentleman!"

"Are you stupid or out of your senses?" asked the doctor angrily. "How can I let him go? Why, he is a convict."

Kirila began crying. "Let him go!"

"Tfoo, queer fellow! What right have I? Am I a jailer or what? They brought him to the hospital for me to treat him, but I have as much right to let him out as I have to put you in prison, silly fellow!"

"But they have shut him up for nothing! He was in prison a year before the trial, and now there is no saying what he is there for. It would have been a different thing if he had murdered someone, let us say, or stolen horses; but as it is, what is it all about?"

"Very likely, but how do I come in?"

"They shut a man up and they don't know themselves what for. He was drunk, your honor, did not know what he was doing, and even hit father on the ear and scratched his own cheek on a branch, and two of our fellows—they wanted some Turkish tobacco, you see—began telling him to go with them and break into the Armenian's shop at night for tobacco. Being drunk, he obeyed them, the fool. They broke the lock, you know, got in, and did no end of mischief; they turned everything upside down, broke the windows and scattered the flour about. They were drunk, that is all one can say! Well, the constable turned up . . . and with one thing and another they took them off to the magistrate. They have been a whole year in prison, and a week ago on the Wednesday, they were all three tried in the town. A soldier stood behind them with a gun . . . people were sworn in. Vaska was less to blame than any, but the gentry decided that he was the ringleader. The other two lads were sent to prison but Vaska to a convict battalion for three years. And what for? One should judge like a Christian!"

"I have nothing to do with it, I tell you again. Go to the authorities."

"I have been already! I've been to the court; I have tried to send a petition— they wouldn't take a petition; I have been to the police captain, and I have been to the examining magistrate, and everyone says, 'It is not my business!' Whose business is it, then? But there is no one above you here in the hospital; you do what you like, your honor."

"You simpleton," sighed the doctor, "once the jury has found him guilty, not the governor, not even the minister, could do anything, let alone the police captain. It's no good your trying to do anything!"

"And who judged him, then?"

"The gentlemen of the jury. . . ."

"They weren't gentlemen, they were our peasants! Andrey Guryev was one; Aloshka Huk was one."

"Well, I am cold talking to you. . . ."

The doctor waved his hand and walked quickly to his own door. Kirila was on the point of following him, but, seeing the door slam, he stopped.

For ten minutes he stood motionless in the middle of the hospital yard, and without putting on his cap stared at the doctor's house, then he heaved a deep sigh, slowly scratched himself, and walked towards the gate.

"To whom am I to go?" he muttered as he came out on to the road. "One says it is not his business, another says it is not his business. Whose business is it, then? No, till you grease their hands you will get nothing out of them. The doctor says that, but he keeps looking all the while at my fist to see whether I am going to give him a blue note. Well, brother, I'll go, if it has to be, to the governor."

Shifting from one foot to the other and continually looking round him in an objectless way, he trudged lazily along the road and was apparently wondering where to go. . . . It was not cold and the snow faintly crunched under his feet. Not more than half a mile in front of him the wretched little district town in which his brother had just been tried lay outstretched on the hill. On the right was the dark prison with its red roof and sentry boxes at the corners; on the left was the big town copse, now covered with the hoar-frost. It was still; only an old man, wearing a woman's short jacket and a huge cap, was walking ahead, coughing and shouting to a cow that he was driving to the town.

"Good day, grandfather," said Kirila, overtaking him.

"Good-day. . . ."

"Are you driving it to the market?"

"No," the old man answered lazily.

"Are you a townsman?"

They got into conversation; Kirila told him what he had come to the hospital for, and what he had been talking about to the doctor.

"The doctor does not know anything about such matters, that is a sure thing," the old man said to him as they were both entering the town; "though he is a gentleman, he is only taught to cure by every means, but to give you real advice, or, let us say, write out a petition for you—that he cannot do. There are special authorities to do that. You have been to the justice of the peace and to the police captain—they are no good for your business either."

"Where am I to go?"

"The permanent member of the rural board is the chief person for peasants' affairs. Go to him, Mr. Sineokov."

"The one who is at Zolotovo?"

"Why, yes, at Zolotovo. He is your chief man. If it is anything that has to do with you peasants even the police captain has no authority against him."

"It's a long way to go, old man. . . . I dare say it's twelve miles and may be more."

"One who needs something will go seventy."

"That is so. . . . Should I send in a petition to him, or what?"

"You will find out there. If you should have a petition, the clerk will write you one quick enough. The permanent member has a clerk."

After parting from the old man Kirila stood still in the middle of the square, thought a little, and walked back out of the town. He made up his mind to go to Zolotovo.

Five days later, as the doctor was on his way home after seeing his patients, he caught sight of Kirila again in his yard. This time the young peasant was not alone, but with a gaunt, very pale old man who nodded his head without ceasing, like a pendulum, and mumbled with his lips.

"Your honor," the old man hissed in his throat, raising his twitching eyebrows, "be merciful! We are poor people, we cannot repay your honor, but if you graciously please, Kiryushka or Vaska can repay you in work. Let them work."

"We will pay with work," said Kirila, and he raised his hand above his head as though he would take an oath. "Let him go! They are starving, they are crying day and night, your honor!"

The young peasant bent a rapid glance on his father, pulled him by the sleeve, and both of them, as at the word of command, fell at the doctor's feet. The latter waved his hand in despair, and, without looking round, walked quickly in at his door.

Enemies

Between nine and ten on a dark September evening the only son of the district doctor, Kirilov, a child of six, called Andrey, died of diphtheria. Just as the doctor's wife sank on her knees by the dead child's bedside and was overwhelmed by the first rush of despair there came a sharp ring at the bell in the entry.

All the servants had been sent out of the house that morning on account of the diphtheria. Kirilov went to open the door just as he was, without his coat on, with his waistcoat unbuttoned, without wiping his wet face or his hands, which were scalded with carbolic. It was dark in the entry and nothing could be distinguished in the man who came in but medium height, a white scarf and a large, extremely pale face, so pale that its entrance seemed to make the passage lighter.

"Is the doctor at home?" the newcomer asked quickly.

"I am at home," answered Kirilov. "What do you want?"

"Oh, it's you? I am very glad," said the stranger in a tone of relief, and he began feeling in the dark for the doctor's hand, found it and squeezed it tightly in his own. "I am very . . . very glad! We are acquainted. My name is Abogin, and I had the honor of meeting you in the summer at Gnutchev's. I am very glad to have found you at home. . . . For God's sake don't refuse to come back with me at once. . . . My wife has been taken dangerously ill. . . . And the carriage is waiting. . . ."

From the voice and gestures of the speaker it could be seen that he was in a state of great excitement. Like a man terrified by a house on fire or a mad dog, he could hardly restrain his rapid breathing and spoke quickly in a shaking voice, and there was a note of unaffected sincerity and childish alarm in his voice. As people always do who are frightened and overwhelmed, he spoke in brief, jerky sentences and uttered a great many unnecessary, irrelevant words.

"I was afraid I might not find you in," he went on. "I was in a perfect agony as I drove here. Put on your things and let us go, for God's sake. . . . This is how it happened. Alexandr Semyonovitch Paptchinsky, whom you know, came to see me. . . . We talked a little and then we sat down to tea; suddenly my wife cried out, clutched at her heart, and fell back on her chair. We carried her to bed and . . .

30

and I rubbed her forehead with ammonia and sprinkled her with water . . . She lay as though she were dead. . . . I am afraid it is aneurysm. . . . Come along . . . her father died of aneurysm."

Kirilov listened and said nothing, as though he did not understand Russian.

When Abogin mentioned again Paptchinsky and his wife's father and once more began feeling in the dark for his hand the doctor shook his head and said apathetically, dragging out each word:

"Excuse me, I cannot come . . . my son died . . . five minutes ago!"

"Is it possible!" whispered Abogin, stepping back a pace. "My God, at what an unlucky moment I have come! A wonderfully unhappy day . . . wonderfully. What a coincidence. . . . It's as though it were on purpose!"

Abogin took hold of the door handle and bowed his head. He was evidently hesitating and did not know what to do—whether to go away or to continue entreating the doctor.

"Listen," he said fervently, catching hold of Kirilov's sleeve. "I well understand your position! God is my witness that I am ashamed of attempting at such a moment to intrude on your attention, but what am I to do? Only think, to whom can I go? There is no other doctor here, you know. For God's sake come! I am not asking you for myself. . . . I am not the patient!"

A silence followed. Kirilov turned his back on Abogin, stood still a moment and slowly walked into the drawing room. Judging from his unsteady, mechanical step, from the attention with which he set straight the fluffy shade on the unlighted lamp in the drawing-room and glanced into a thick book lying on the table, at that instant he had no intention, no desire, was thinking of nothing and most likely did not remember that there was a stranger in the entry. The twilight and stillness of the drawing room seemed to increase his numbness. Going out of the drawing-room into his study he raised his right foot higher than was necessary, and felt for the doorposts with his hands, and as he did so there was an air of perplexity about his whole figure as though he were in somebody else's house, or were drunk for the first time in his life and were now abandoning himself with surprise to the new sensation. A broad streak of light stretched across the bookcase on one wall of the study; this light came together with the close, heavy smell of carbolic and ether from the door into the bedroom, which stood a little way open. . . . The doctor sank into a low chair in front of the table; for a minute he stared drowsily at his books, which lay with the light on them, then got up and went into the bedroom.

Here in the bedroom reigned a dead silence. Everything to the smallest detail was eloquent of the storm that had been passed through, of exhaustion and everything was at rest. A candle standing among a crowd of bottles, boxes, and pots on a stool and a big lamp on the chest of drawers threw a brilliant light over all the room. On the bed under the window lay a boy with open eyes and a look of wonder on his face. He did not move, but his open eyes seemed every moment growing darker and sinking further into his head. The mother was kneeling by the bed with her arms on his body and her head hidden in the bed-clothes. Like the child, she did not stir; but what throbbing life was suggested in the curves of her body and in her arms! She leaned against the bed with all her being, pressing against it greedily with all her might, as though she were afraid of disturbing the peaceful and comfortable attitude she had found at last for her exhausted body. The bedclothes, the rags and bowls, the splashes of water on the floor, the little paintbrushes and spoons thrown down here and there, the white bottle of lime water, the very air, heavy and stifling—were all hushed and seemed plunged in repose.

The doctor stopped close to his wife, thrust his hands in his trouser pockets, and slanting his head on one side fixed his eyes on his son. His face bore an expression of indifference, and only from the drops that glittered on his beard it could be seen that he had just been crying.

That repellent horror which is thought of when we speak of death was absent from the room. In the numbness of everything, in the mother's attitude, in the indifference on the doctor's face there was something that attracted and touched the heart, that subtle almost elusive beauty of human sorrow which men will not for a long time learn to understand and describe, and which it seems only music can convey. There was a feeling of beauty, too, in the austere stillness. Kirilov and his wife were silent and not weeping, as though besides the bitterness of their loss they were conscious, too, of all the tragedy of their position; just as once their youth had passed away, so now together with this boy their right to have children had gone for ever to all eternity! The doctor was forty-four, his hair was grey and he looked like an old man; his faded and invalid wife was thirty-five. Andrey was not merely the only child, but also the last child.

In contrast to his wife the doctor belonged to the class of people who at times of spiritual suffering feel a craving for movement. After standing for five minutes by his wife, he walked, raising his right foot high, from the bedroom into a little room which was half filled up by a big sofa; from there he went into the kitchen. After wandering by the stove and the cook's bed he bent down and went by a little door into the passage.

There he saw again the white scarf and the white face.

"At last," sighed Abogin, reaching towards the door-handle. "Let us go, please."

The doctor started, glanced at him, and remembered. . . .

"Why, I have told you already that I can't go!" he said, growing more animated. "How strange!"

"Doctor, I am not a stone, I fully understand your position. . . . I feel for you," Abogin said in an imploring voice, laying his hand on his scarf. "But I am not asking you for myself. My wife is dying. If you had heard that cry, if you had seen her face, you would understand my pertinacity. My God, I thought you had gone to get ready! Doctor, time is precious. Let us go, I entreat you."

"I cannot go," said Kirilov emphatically, and he took a step into the drawing-room.

Abogin followed him and caught hold of his sleeve.

"You are in sorrow, I understand. But I'm not asking you to a case of tooth-ache or to a consultation, but to save a human life!" he went on entreating like a beggar. "Life comes before any personal sorrow! Come, I ask for courage, for hero-ism! For the love of humanity!"

"Humanity—that cuts both ways," Kirilov said irritably. "In the name of hu-manity I beg you not to take me. And how queer it is, really! I can hardly stand and you talk to me about humanity! I am fit for nothing just now. . . . Nothing will induce me to go, and I can't leave my wife alone. No, no. . . ."

Kirilov waved his hands and staggered back.

"And . . . and don't ask me," he went on in a tone of alarm. "Excuse me. By No. XIII of the regulations I am obliged to go and you have the right to drag me by my collar . . . drag me if you like, but . . . I am not fit . . . I can't even speak . . . excuse me."

"There is no need to take that tone to me, doctor!" said Abogin, again taking the doctor by his sleeve. "What do I care about No. XIII! To force you against your will I have no right whatever. If you will, come; if you will not—God for-give you; but I am not appealing to your will, but to your feelings. A young woman is dying. You were just speaking of the death of your son. Who should under-stand my horror if not you?"

Abogin's voice quivered with emotion; that quiver and his tone were far more persuasive than his words. Abogin was sincere, but it was remarkable that what-ever he said his words sounded stilted, soulless, and inappropriately flowery, and even seemed an outrage on the atmosphere of the doctor's home and on the woman who was somewhere dying. He felt himself, and so, afraid of not being understood, did his utmost to put softness and tenderness into his voice so that the sincerity of his tone might prevail if his words did not. As a rule, however fine and deep a phrase may be, it only affects the indifferent, and cannot fully sat-isfy those who are happy or unhappy; that is why dumbness is most often the highest expression of happiness or unhappiness; lovers understand each other better when they are silent, and a fervent, passionate speech delivered by the grave only touches outsiders, while to the widow and children of the dead man it seems cold and trivial.

Kirilov stood in silence. When Abogin uttered a few more phrases concerning the noble calling of a doctor, self-sacrifice, and so on, the doctor asked sullenly: "Is it far?"

"Something like eight or nine miles. I have capital horses, doctor! I give you my word of honor that I will get you there and back in an hour. Only one hour."

These words had more effect on Kirilov than the appeals to humanity or the noble calling of the doctor. He thought a moment and said with a sigh: "Very well, let us go!"

He went rapidly with a more certain step to his study, and afterwards came back in a long frock-coat. Abogin, greatly relieved, fidgeted round him and scraped with his feet as he helped him on with his overcoat, and went out of the house with him.

It was dark out of doors, though lighter than in the entry. The tall, stooping figure of the doctor, with his long, narrow beard and aquiline nose, stood out distinctly in the darkness. Abogin's big head and the little student's cap that barely covered it could be seen now as well as his pale face. The scarf showed white only in front, behind it was hidden by his long hair.

"Believe me, I know how to appreciate your generosity," Abogin muttered as he helped the doctor into the carriage. "We shall get there quickly. Drive as fast as you can, Luka, there's a good fellow! Please!"

The coachman drove rapidly. At first there was a row of indistinct buildings that stretched alongside the hospital yard; it was dark everywhere except for a bright light from a window that gleamed through the fence into the furthest part of the yard while three windows of the upper story of the hospital looked paler than the surrounding air. Then the carriage drove into dense shadow; here there was the smell of dampness and mushrooms, and the sound of rustling trees; the crows, awakened by the noise of the wheels, stirred among the foliage and uttered prolonged plaintive cries as though they knew the doctor's son was dead and that Abogin's wife was ill. Then came glimpses of separate trees, of bushes; a pond, on which great black shadows were slumbering, gleamed with a sullen light—and the carriage rolled over a smooth level ground. The clamor of the crows sounded dimly far away and soon ceased altogether.

Kirilov and Abogin were silent almost all the way. Only once Abogin heaved a deep sigh and muttered:

"It's an agonizing state! One never loves those who are near one so much as when one is in danger of losing them."

And when the carriage slowly drove over the river, Kirilov started all at once as though the splash of the water had frightened him, and made a movement.

"Listen—let me go," he said miserably. "I'll come to you later. I must just send my assistant to my wife. She is alone, you know!"

Abogin did not speak. The carriage swaying from side to side and crunching over the stones drove up the sandy bank and rolled on its way. Kirilov moved restlessly and looked about him in misery. Behind them in the dim light of the stars the road could be seen and the riverside willows vanishing into the darkness. On the right lay a plain as uniform and as boundless as the sky; here and there in the distance, probably on the peat marshes, dim lights were glimmering. On the left, parallel with the road, ran a hill tufted with small bushes, and above the hill stood motionless a big, red half-moon, slightly veiled with mist and encircled by tiny clouds, which seemed to be looking round at it from all sides and watching that it did not go away.

In all nature there seemed to be a feeling of hopelessness and pain. The earth, like a ruined woman sitting alone in a dark room and trying not to think of the past, was brooding over memories of spring and summer and apathetically waiting for the inevitable winter. Wherever one looked, on all sides, nature seemed like a dark, infinitely deep, cold pit from which neither Kirilov nor Abogin nor the red half-moon could escape. . . .

The nearer the carriage got to its goal the more impatient Abogin became. He kept moving, leaping up, looking over the coachmen's shoulder. And when at last the carriage stopped before the entrance, which was elegantly curtained with striped linen, and when he looked at the lighted windows of the second story there was an audible catch in his breath.

"If anything happens . . . I shall not survive it," he said, going into the hall with the doctor, and rubbing his hands in agitation. "But there is no commotion, so everything must be going well so far," he added, listening in the stillness.

There was no sound in the hall of steps or voices and all the house seemed asleep in spite of the lighted windows. Now the doctor and Abogin, who till then had been in darkness, could see each other clearly. The doctor was tall and stooped, was untidily dressed and not good-looking. There was an unpleasantly harsh, morose, and unfriendly look about his lips, thick as a Negro's, his aquiline nose, and listless, apathetic eyes. His unkempt head and sunken temples, the premature greyness of his long, narrow beard through which his chin was visible, the pale grey hue of his skin and his careless, uncouth manners—the harshness of all this was suggestive of years of poverty, of ill fortune, of weariness with life and with men. Looking at his frigid figure one could hardly believe that this man had a wife, that he was capable of weeping over his child. Abogin presented a very different appearance. He was a thickset, sturdy-looking, fair man with a big head and large, soft features; he was elegantly dressed in the very latest fashion. In his carriage, his closely buttoned coat, his long hair, and his face there was a suggestion of something generous, leonine; he walked with his head erect and his chest squared, he spoke in an agreeable baritone, and there was a shade of refined almost feminine elegance in the manner in which he took off his scarf and smoothed his hair. Even his paleness and the childlike terror with which he looked up at the stairs as he took off his coat did not detract from his dignity nor diminish the air of sleekness, health, and aplomb, which characterized his whole figure.

"There is nobody and no sound," he said going up the stairs. "There is no commotion. God grant all is well."

He led the doctor through the hall into a big drawing-room where there was a black piano and a chandelier in a white cover; from there they both went into a very snug, pretty little drawing-room full of an agreeable, rosy twilight.

"Well, sit down here, doctor and I . . . will be back directly. I will go and have a look and prepare them."

Kirilov was left alone. The luxury of the drawing-room, the agreeably subdued light and his own presence in the stranger's unfamiliar house, which had something of the character of an adventure, did not apparently affect him. He sat in a low chair and scrutinized his hands, which were burnt with carbolic. He only caught a passing glimpse of the bright red lamp-shade and the violoncello case, and glancing in the direction where the clock was ticking he noticed a stuffed wolf as substantial and sleek-looking as Abogin himself.

It was quiet. . . . Somewhere far away in the adjoining rooms someone uttered a loud exclamation: "Ah!" There was a clang of a glass door, probably of a cupboard, and again all was still. After waiting five minutes Kirilov left off scrutinizing his hands and raised his eyes to the door by which Abogin had vanished.

In the doorway stood Abogin, but he was not the same as when he had gone out. The look of sleekness and refined elegance had disappeared—his face, his hands, his attitude were contorted by a revolting expression of something between horror and agonizing physical pain. His nose, his lips, his moustache, all his features were moving and seemed trying to tear themselves from his face, his eyes looked as though they were laughing with agony. . . .

Abogin took a heavy stride into the drawing room, bent forward, moaned, and shook his fists.

"She has deceived me," he cried, with a strong emphasis on the second syllable of the verb. "Deceived me, gone away. She fell ill and sent me for the doctor only to run away with that clown Paptchinsky! My God!"

Abogin took a heavy step towards the doctor, held out his soft white fists in his face, and shaking them went on yelling:

"Gone away! Deceived me! But why this deception? My God! My God! What need of this dirty, scoundrelly trick, this diabolical, snakish farce? What have I done to her? Gone away!"

Tears gushed from his eyes. He turned on one foot and began pacing up and down the drawing room. Now in his short coat, his fashionable narrow trousers which made his legs look disproportionately slim, with his big head and long mane he was extremely like a lion. A gleam of curiosity came into the apathetic face of the doctor. He got up and looked at Abogin.

"Excuse me, where is the patient?" he said.

"The patient! The patient!" cried Abogin, laughing, crying, and still brandishing his fists. "She is not ill, but accursed! The baseness! The vileness! The devil himself could not have imagined anything more loathsome! She sent me off that she might run away with a buffoon, a dull-witted clown, an Alphonse! Oh God, better she had died! I cannot bear it! I cannot bear it!"

The doctor drew himself up. His eyes blinked and filled with tears, his narrow beard began moving to right and to left together with his jaw.

"Allow me to ask what's the meaning of this?" he asked, looking round him with curiosity. "My child is dead, my wife is in grief alone in the whole house. . . . I myself can scarcely stand up, I have not slept for three nights. . . . And here I am forced to play a part in some vulgar farce, to play the part of a stage property! I don't . . . don't understand it!"

Abogin unclenched one fist, flung a crumpled note on the floor and stamped on it as though it were an insect he wanted to crush.

"And I didn't see, didn't understand," he said through his clenched teeth, brandishing one fist before his face with an expression as though some one had trodden on his corns. "I did not notice that he came every day! I did not notice that he came today in a closed carriage! What did he come in a closed carriage for? And I did not see it! Noodle!"

"I don't understand . . ." muttered the doctor. "Why, what's the meaning of it? Why, it's an outrage on personal dignity, a mockery of human suffering! It's incredible. . . . It's the first time in my life I have had such an experience!"

With the dull surprise of a man who has only just realized that he has been bitterly insulted, the doctor shrugged his shoulders, flung wide his arms, and not knowing what to do or to say sank helplessly into a chair.

"If you have ceased to love me and love another—so be it; but why this deceit, why this vulgar, treacherous trick?" Abogin said in a tearful voice. "What is the object of it? And what is there to justify it? And what have I done to you? Listen, doctor," he said hotly, going up to Kirilov. "You have been the involuntary witness of my misfortune and I am not going to conceal the truth from you. I swear that I loved the woman, loved her devotedly, like a slave! I have sacrificed everything for her; I have quarreled with my own people, I have given up the service and music, I have forgiven her what I could not have forgiven my own mother or sister. I have never looked askance at her. . . . I have never gainsaid her in any-thing. Why this deception? I do not demand love, but why this loathsome du-plicity? If she did not love me, why did she not say so openly, honestly, especially as she knows my views on the subject?"

With tears in his eyes, trembling all over, Abogin opened his heart to the doc-tor with perfect sincerity. He spoke warmly, pressing both hands on his heart, exposing the secrets of his private life without the faintest hesitation, and even seemed to be glad that at last these secrets were no longer pent up in his breast. If he had talked in this way for an hour or two, and opened his heart, he would undoubtedly have felt better. Who knows, if the doctor had listened to him and had sympathized with him like a friend, he might perhaps, as often happens, have reconciled himself to his trouble without protest, without doing anything need-less and absurd. . . . But what happened was quite different. While Abogin was speaking the outraged doctor perceptibly changed. The indifference and wonder on his face gradually gave way to an expression of bitter resentment, indignation, and anger. The features of his face became even harsher, coarser, and more un-pleasant. When Abogin held out before his eyes the photograph of a young woman with a handsome face as cold and expressionless as a nun's and asked him whether, looking at that face, one could conceive that it was capable of duplicity, the doc-tor suddenly flew out, and with flashing eyes, said, rudely rapping out each word:

"What are you telling me all this for? I have no desire to hear it! I have no desire to!" he shouted and brought his fist down on the table. "I don't want your vulgar secrets! Damnation take them! Don't dare to tell me of such vulgar do-ings! Do you consider that I have not been insulted enough already? That I am a flunkey whom you can insult without restraint? Is that it?"

Abogin staggered back from Kirilov and stared at him in amazement.

"Why did you bring me here?" the doctor went on, his beard quivering. "If you are so puffed up with good living that you go and get married and then act a farce like this, how do I come in? What have I to do with your love affairs? Leave me in peace! Go on squeezing money out of the poor in your gentlemanly way. Make a display of humane ideas, play (the doctor looked sideways at the violon-cello case), play the bassoon and the trombone, grow as fat as capons, but don't dare to insult personal dignity! If you cannot respect it, you might at least spare it your attention!"

"Excuse me, what does all this mean?" Abogin asked, flushing red.

"It means that it's base and low to play with people like this! I am a doctor; you look upon doctors and people generally who work and don't stink of per-fume and prostitution as your menials and *mauvais ton;* well, you may look upon them so, but no one has given you the right to treat a man who is suffering as a stage property!"

"How dare you say that to me!" Abogin said quietly, and his face began working again, and this time unmistakably from the anger.

"No, how dared you, knowing of my sorrow, bring me here to listen to these vulgarities!" shouted the doctor, and he again banged on the table with his fist. "Who has given you the right to make a mockery of another man's sorrow?"

"You have taken leave of your senses," shouted Abogin. "It is ungenerous. I am intensely unhappy myself and . . . and . . ."

"Unhappy!" said the doctor, with a smile of contempt. "Don't utter that word, it does not concern you. The spendthrift who cannot raise a loan calls himself unhappy, too. The capon, sluggish from over-feeding, is unhappy, too. Worthless people!"

"Sir, you forget yourself," shrieked Abogin. "For saying things like that . . . people are thrashed! Do you understand?"

Abogin hurriedly felt in his side pocket, pulled out a pocket book, and extracting two notes flung them on the table.

"Here is the fee for your visit," he said, his nostrils dilating. "You are paid."

"How dare you offer me money?" shouted the doctor and he brushed the notes off the table on to the floor. "An insult cannot be paid for in money!"

Abogin and the doctor stood face to face, and in their wrath continued flinging undeserved insults at each other. I believe that never in their lives, even in delirium, had they uttered so much that was unjust, cruel, and absurd. The egoism of the unhappy was conspicuous in both. The unhappy are egoistic, spiteful, unjust, cruel, and less capable of understanding each other than fools. Unhappiness does not bring people together but draws them apart, and even where one would fancy people should be united by the similarity of their sorrow, far more injustice and cruelty is generated than in comparatively placid surroundings.

"Kindly let me go home!" shouted the doctor, breathing hard.

Abogin rang the bell sharply. When no one came to answer the bell he rang again and angrily flung the bell on the floor; it fell on the carpet with a muffled sound, and uttered a plaintive note as though at the point of death. A footman came in.

"Where have you been hiding yourself, the devil take you?" His master flew at him, clenching his fists. "Where were you just now? Go and tell them to bring the Victoria round for this gentleman, and order the closed carriage to be got ready for me. Stay," he cried as the footman turned to go out. "I won't have a single traitor in the house by tomorrow! Away with you all! I will engage fresh servants! Reptiles!"

Abogin and the doctor remained in silence waiting for the carriage. The first regained his expression of sleekness and his refined elegance. He paced up and down the room, tossed his head elegantly, and was evidently meditating on something. His anger had not cooled, but he tried to appear not to notice his enemy. . . .

The doctor stood, leaning with one hand on the edge of the table, and looked at Abogin with that profound and somewhat cynical, ugly contempt only to be found in the eyes of sorrow and indigence when they are confronted with well-nourished comfort and elegance.

When a little later the doctor got into the Victoria and drove off there was still a look of contempt in his eyes. It was dark, much darker than it had been an hour before. The red half-moon had sunk behind the hill and the clouds that had been guarding it lay in dark patches near the stars. The carriage with red lamps rattled along the road and soon overtook the doctor. It was Abogin driving off to protest, to do absurd things. . . .

All the way home the doctor thought not of his wife, nor of his Andrey, but of Abogin and the people in the house he had just left. His thoughts were unjust and inhumanly cruel. He condemned Abogin and his wife and Paptchinsky and all who lived in rosy, subdued light among sweet perfumes, and all the way home he hated and despised them till his head ached. And a firm conviction concerning those people took shape in his mind.

Time will pass and Kirilov's sorrow will pass, but that conviction, unjust and unworthy of the human heart, will not pass, but will remain in the doctor's mind to the grave.

The Examining Magistrate

A district doctor and an examining magistrate were driving one fine spring day to an inquest. The examining magistrate, a man of five and thirty, looked dreamily at the horses and said:

"There is a great deal that is enigmatic and obscure in nature; and even in everyday life, doctor, one must often come upon phenomena which are absolutely incapable of explanation. I know, for instance, of several strange, mysterious deaths, the cause of which only spiritualists and mystics will undertake to explain; a clear-headed man can only lift up his hands in perplexity. For example, I know of a highly cultured lady who foretold her own death and died without any apparent reason on the very day she had predicted. She said that she would die on a certain day, and she did die."

"There's no effect without a cause," said the doctor. "If there's a death there must be a cause for it. But as for predicting it there's nothing very marvelous in that. All our ladies—all our females, in fact—have a turn for prophecies and presentiments."

"Just so, but my lady, doctor, was quite a special case. There was nothing like the ladies' or other females' presentiments about her prediction and her death. She was a young woman, healthy and clever, with no superstitions of any sort. She had such clear, intelligent, honest eyes; an open, sensible face with a faint, typically Russian look of mockery in her eyes and on her lips. There was nothing of the fine lady or of the female about her, except—if you like—her beauty! She was graceful, elegant as that birch tree; she had wonderful hair. That she may be intelligible to you, I will add, too, that she was a person of the most infectious gaiety and carelessness and that intelligent, good sort of frivolity which is only found in good-natured, lighthearted people with brains. Can one talk of mysticism, spiritualism, a turn for presentiment, or anything of that sort, in this case? She used to laugh at all that."

The doctor's chaise stopped by a well. The examining magistrate and the doctor drank some water, stretched, and waited for the coachman to finish watering the horses.

"Well, what did the lady die of?" asked the doctor when the chaise was rolling along the road again.

"She died in a strange way. One fine day her husband went in to her and said that it wouldn't be amiss to sell their old coach before the spring and to buy something rather newer and lighter instead, and that it might be as well to change the left trace horse and to put Bobtchinsky (that was the name of one of her husband's horses) in the shafts.

"His wife listened to him and said:

"'Do as you think best, but it makes no difference to me now. Before the summer I shall be in the cemetery.'

"Her husband, of course, shrugged his shoulders and smiled.

"'I am not joking,' she said. 'I tell you in earnest that I shall soon be dead.'

"'What do you mean by soon?'

"'Directly after my confinement. I shall bear my child and die.'

"The husband attached no significance to these words. He did not believe in presentiments of any sort, and he knew that ladies in an interesting condition are apt to be fanciful and to give way to gloomy ideas generally. A day later his wife spoke to him again of dying immediately after her confinement, and then every day she spoke of it and he laughed and called her a silly woman, a fortuneteller, a crazy creature. Her approaching death became an *idee fixe* with his wife. When her husband would not listen to her she would go into the kitchen and talk of her death to the nurse and the cook.

"'I haven't long to live now, nurse,' she would say. 'As soon as my confinement is over I shall die. I did not want to die so early, but it seems it's my fate.'

"The nurse and the cook were in tears, of course. Sometimes the priest's wife or some lady from a neighbouring estate would come and see her and she would take them aside and open her soul to them, always harping on the same subject, her approaching death. She spoke gravely with an unpleasant smile, even with an angry face which would not allow any contradiction. She had been smart and fashionable in her dress, but now in view of her approaching death she became slovenly; she did not read, she did not laugh, she did not dream aloud. What was more she drove with her aunt to the cemetery and selected a spot for her tomb. Five days before her confinement she made her will. And all this, bear in mind, was done in the best of health, without the faintest hint of illness or danger. A confinement is a difficult affair and sometimes fatal, but in the case of which I am telling you every indication was favorable, and there was absolutely nothing to be afraid of. Her husband was sick of the whole business at last. He lost his temper one day at dinner and asked her:

"'Listen, Natasha, when is there going to be an end of this silliness?'

"'It's not silliness, I am in earnest.'

"'Nonsense, I advise you to give over being silly that you may not feel ashamed of it afterwards.'

"Well, the confinement came. The husband got the very best midwife from the town. It was his wife's first confinement, but it could not have gone better. When it was all over she asked to look at her baby. She looked at it and said:

"'Well, now I can die.'

"She said good-bye, shut her eyes, and half an hour later gave up her soul to God. She was fully conscious up to the last moment. Anyway, when they gave her milk instead of water she whispered softly:

"'Why are you giving me milk instead of water?'

"So that is what happened. She died as she predicted."

The examining magistrate paused, gave a sigh and said:

"Come, explain why she died. I assure you on my honor, this is not invented, it's a fact."

The doctor looked at the sky meditatively.

"You ought to have had an inquest on her," he said.

"Why?"

"Why, to find out the cause of her death. She didn't die because she had predicted it. She poisoned herself most probably."

The examining magistrate turned quickly, facing the doctor, and screwing up his eyes, asked:

"And from what do you conclude that she poisoned herself?"

"I don't conclude it, but I assume it. Was she on good terms with her husband?"

"H'm, not altogether. There had been misunderstandings soon after their marriage. There were unfortunate circumstances. She had found her husband on one occasion with a lady. She soon forgave him however."

"And which came first, her husband's infidelity or her idea of dying?"

The examining magistrate looked attentively at the doctor as though he were trying to imagine why he put that question.

"Excuse me," he said, not quite immediately.

"Let me try and remember." The examining magistrate took off his hat and rubbed his forehead.

"Yes, yes . . . it was very shortly after that incident that she began talking of death. Yes, yes."

"Well, there, do you see? . . . In all probability it was at that time that she made up her mind to poison herself, but, as most likely she did not want to kill her child also, she put it off till after her confinement."

"Not likely, not likely! . . . it's impossible. She forgave him at the time."

"That she forgave it quickly means that she had something bad in her mind. Young wives do not forgive quickly."

The examining magistrate gave a forced smile, and, to conceal his too noticeable agitation, began lighting a cigarette.

"Not likely, not likely," he went on. "No notion of anything of the sort being possible ever entered into my head. . . . And besides . . . he was not so much to blame as it seems. . . . He was unfaithful to her in rather a queer way, with no desire to be; he came home at night somewhat elevated, wanted to make love to somebody, his wife was in an interesting condition. Then he came across a lady who had come to stay for three days—damnation take her—an empty-headed creature, silly and not good-looking. It couldn't be reckoned as an infidelity. His wife looked at it in that way herself and soon . . . forgave it. Nothing more was said about it."

"People don't die without a reason," said the doctor.

"That is so, of course, but all the same . . . I cannot admit that she poisoned herself. But it is strange that the idea has never struck me before! And no one thought of it! Everyone was astonished that her prediction had come to pass, and the idea . . . of such a death was far from their mind. And indeed, it cannot be that she poisoned herself! No!"

The examining magistrate pondered. The thought of the woman who had died so strangely haunted him all through the inquest. As he noted down what the doctor dictated to him he moved his eyebrows gloomily and rubbed his forehead.

"And are there really poisons that kill one in a quarter of an hour, gradually, without any pain?" he asked the doctor while the latter was opening the skull.

"Yes, there are. Morphia, for instance."

"H'm, strange. I remember she used to keep something of the sort. . . . But it could hardly be."

On the way back the examining magistrate looked exhausted, he kept nervously biting his moustache, and was unwilling to talk.

"Let us go a little way on foot," he said to the doctor. "I am tired of sitting."

After walking about a hundred paces, the examining magistrate seemed to the doctor to be overcome with fatigue, as though he had been climbing up a high mountain. He stopped and, looking at the doctor with a strange look in his eyes, as though he were drunk, said:

"My God, if your theory is correct, why it's . . . it was cruel, inhuman! She poisoned herself to punish someone else! Why, was the sin so great? Oh, my God! And why did you make me a present of this damnable idea, doctor!"

The examining magistrate clutched at his head in despair, and went on:

"What I have told you was about my own wife, about myself. Oh, my God! I was to blame, I wounded her, but can it have been easier to die than to forgive? That's typical feminine logic—cruel, merciless logic. Oh, even then when she was living she was cruel! I recall it all now! It's all clear to me now!"

As the examining magistrate talked he shrugged his shoulders, then clutched at his head. He got back into the carriage, then walked again. The new idea the doctor had imparted to him seemed to have overwhelmed him, to have poisoned him; he was distracted, shattered in body and soul, and when he got back to the town he said good-bye to the doctor, declining to stay to dinner though he had promised the doctor the evening before to dine with him.

An Awkward Business

Grigory Ivanovich Ovchinnikov, a Zemstvo doctor, was a nervous man of about thirty-five, in poor health. He was known to his colleagues by his short papers on medical statistics and for his keen interest in so-called "problems of daily life." One morning he was making the rounds of the hospital of which he was in charge, followed, as usual, by his *feldscher* (medical assistant), Mikhail Zakharych, an elderly man with a fleshy face, greasy hair plastered down over his scalp, and one earring.

No sooner did the doctor start his rounds than one trifling circumstance began to seem very suspicious to him: the *feldscher's* waistcoat was creased and was continually riding up, in spite of the fact that he kept pulling at it and straightening it. His shirt, too, was mussed and rumpled; there was white fluff on his long, black jacket, on his trousers, and even on his tie. Obviously, the *feldscher* had slept in his clothes all night, and, to judge by his expression as he pulled at his waistcoat and straightened his tie, he felt uncomfortable in his clothes.

The doctor looked at him closely and grasped the situation. The *feldscher* was steady on his feet, he answered questions coherently, but the dull and sullen expression of his face, his lusterless eyes, his jerking neck and trembling hands, his disordered clothes, above all, the strenuous efforts he was making to conceal his condition—all pointed to the fact that he had just tumbled out of bed, that he had not had enough sleep, and that he had not got over the effects of the previous night's drinking-bout. He was in the grip of an excruciating hangover and apparently very much displeased with himself.

The doctor, who disliked the *feldscher,* and had his reasons for it, felt a strong desire to say to him: "I see you're drunk!" All at once he was overcome by disgust for the waistcoat, the long jacket, the ring in the fleshy ear, but he controlled his irritation and said gently and politely, as usual:

"Did Gerasim get his milk?

"Yes, sir. . . ." Mikhail Zakharych replied, also in a mild tone.

As the doctor talked to Gerasim, he glanced at the temperature chart and was overcome by a new access of loathing. He checked himself, but lost control and asked rudely, choking on the words:

"Why isn't the temperature noted?"

"But it is, sir!" said Mikhail Zakharych quietly; then, glancing at the chart and discovering that the temperature had indeed not been noted, he shrugged his shoulders with an air of confusion and mumbled:

"I don't know, sir, Nadezhda Osipovna must have . . ."

"Last night's temperature wasn't noted, either!" the doctor went on. "All you do is get drunk, damn you! Even now you're as drunk as a cobbler! Where is Nadezhda Osipovna?"

Nadezhda Osipovna, the midwife, was not in the ward, although it was her duty to be present at the dressings every morning. The doctor looked around, and it seemed to him that the ward had not been tidied up, that everything was at sixes and sevens, that nothing had been done that should have been done and that everything was messy, crumpled, covered with fluff, like the *feldscher's* loathsome waistcoat, and he was filled with a desire to tear off his white apron, to rant, to throw everything up, to send it to the devil and get out. But he mastered himself and continued his rounds.

After Gerasim came a patient who had inflammation of the cellular tissue of the entire right arm. He needed a dressing. The doctor sat down on a stool in front of him and busied himself with the arm.

"Last night they must have had a gay time at a birthday celebration. . . ." he thought to himself, slowly removing the bandage. "Wait, I'll show you a birthday! Although, what can I do? I can do nothing."

He felt an abscess on the red, swollen arm, and said:

"A scalpel!"

Mikhail Zakharych, who was at pains to prove that he was steady on his pins and as fit as a fiddle, dashed from where he was standing and quickly handed over a scalpel.

"Not this! A new one," said the doctor.

The assistant walked mincingly across to the stool on which stood the box with supplies and instruments and began hastily rummaging in it. He kept on whispering to the nurses, noisily moving the box about on the stool, and twice he dropped something. Meanwhile, the doctor sat there, waiting, and felt a physical sense of irritation at the whispering and the other noise.

"Well?" he demanded. "You must have left them downstairs. . . ."

The *feldscher* ran up to him and handed him two scalpels, and in doing so carelessly breathed in the doctor's face.

"Not these," the doctor snapped irritably. "I told you plainly: give me a new one. Never mind, go and get some sleep; you reek like a pothouse. You can't be trusted."

"What other kind of knives do you want?" asked the *feldscher,* in a tone of irritation and with a lazy shrug of his shoulders.

He was annoyed with himself and ashamed because all the patients and nurses were staring at him, and to hide the fact that he was ashamed, he forced a smirk and repeated:

"What other kind of knives do you want?"

The doctor felt tears rising to his eyes and was conscious of a tremor in his fingers. He made another effort to control himself and brought out in a shaking voice:

"Go and sleep it out! I don't want to talk to a drunk. . . ."

"You can call me to account only for cause," said the assistant, "and if I've had a drop, well, nobody has the right to throw it up to me. I'm on duty, ain't I? What more do you want? I'm on duty, ain't I?"

The doctor leapt to his feet and, without realizing what he was doing, swung his fist and hit the *feldscher* with all his might. He might not understand why he had done it, but he felt great pleasure because the blow landed smack in the *feldscher's* face, and that solid citizen, a family man, a churchgoer, substantial, self-respecting, staggered, bounced like a ball and sat down on a stool. The doctor had a passionate urge to hit out again, but when he saw the pale, alarmed faces of the nurses clustered about that hateful countenance, his pleasure died away, he waved his hand in a gesture of desperation and ran out of the ward.

In the courtyard he encountered Nadezhda Osipovna, an unmarried woman about twenty-seven years old, with a sallow complexion and her hair loose over her shoulders, who was on her way to the hospital. The skirt of her pink cotton dress was narrow, and so she walked mincingly. Her dress rustled, she jerked her shoulders in time with her steps and tossed her head as if she were mentally humming a gay tune.

"Aha, the siren!" the doctor said to himself, recalling that in the hospital they called the midwife a siren to tease her. And he took pleasure in the thought that he was about to give a piece of his mind to this mincing, self-infatuated, would-be dressy creature.

"Where on earth have you been?" he exclaimed, as they approached each other. "Why aren't you in the hospital? The temperatures haven't been recorded, everything's at sixes and sevens, the *feldscher* is drunk, you sleep till noon! . . . You'd better look for another position! You're fired!"

Having reached his apartment, the doctor tore off his white apron and the towel which served him as a belt, angrily tossed both of them into a corner, and began pacing the room.

"God, what people, what people!" he groaned. "They're no help, they just get in the way of the work! I haven't the strength to go on! I can't do it. I'm getting out."

His heart was pounding, he was trembling all over, and he felt like bursting into tears. He tried to quiet himself with the thought that he had been in the right, and that it was a good thing that he had struck the *feldscher*. In the first place, reflected the doctor, it was abominable that the hospital should have engaged a man not on his own merits but owing to the intercession of his aunt, who was employed as a nursemaid by the chairman of the Zemstvo board. It was disgusting to see how this influential nanny, when she drove to the hospital for treatment, behaved as though she were at home and refused to wait her turn. The *feldscher* was badly trained, knew very little, and did not understand what he had learned. He drank, was insolent, untidy, accepted bribes from the patients, and secretly sold the medicines supplied free by the Zemstvo. Moreover, everyone knew that he practiced medicine on the quiet, and treated young men from the town for unmentionable diseases, using remedies of his own concoction. It would have not have been so bad if he had simply been a quack, of whom there were plenty, but no—he was a quack who believed in himself, a quack who was furtively in revolt. Behind the doctor's back he cupped and bled dispensary patients, he assisted at operations without having washed his hands, he always examined wounds with a dirty probe. All this was sufficient to show how profoundly and completely he despised the doctors' medicine with its rules and regulations.

When at last his fingers were steady again, the doctor sat down at his desk and wrote a letter to the chairman of the board:

Esteemed Lev Trofimovich!
If on receipt of this note your board does not discharge feldscher *Mikhail Zakharych Smirnovsky, and will not grant me the right to choose my feldscher, I shall regretfully be forced to resign as a physician of the N. hospital and request you to secure someone to succeed me. Please remember me to Lubov Fyodorovna and to Yus. Respectfully,*
G. Ovchinnikov.

Having reread this letter, the doctor decided that it was too short and not sufficiently formal. Besides, the mention of Lubov Fyodorovna and of Yus (the nickname of the chairman's younger son) was hardly appropriate in a business letter dealing with an official matter.

"The devil, why bring in Yus?" the doctor said to himself, tore the letter to bits, and started thinking of another. "Dear Sir," he began. Through the open window he could see a flock of ducks with their young. Waddling and stumbling, they were hurrying down the road, apparently on their way to the pond. One duckling picked up a piece of gut that was lying on the ground, tried to swallow it, choked on it and raised an alarmed squeaking. Another duckling ran up, pulled the gut out of its beak and choked on the thing too. . . . At some distance from the fence, in the lacy shadow cast on the grass by the young lindens, the cook Darya was wandering about, picking sorrel for a vegetable soup. . . . Voices were heard. . . .

Zot, the coachman, with a bridle in his hand, and Manuilo, the hospital attendant, wearing a dirty apron, were standing by the shed, chatting and laughing.

"They are talking about my having struck the *feldscher*. . . ." thought the doctor. "Before the day is over the whole district will know about this scandal. . . . And so: 'Dear Sir! If your board does not discharge . . . .'"

The doctor knew very well that under no circumstance would the board dismiss him rather than the *feldscher,* that it would let every *feldscher* in the whole district go, rather than lose such an excellent man as Doctor Ouchinnikov. Certainly, as soon as Lev Tromfimovich got the letter he would drive up in his troika and commence: "What's this that you've taken into your head, old man? My dear fellow! What is it? In Christ's name! Why? What's the matter? Where is he? Fetch the blackguard here! He must be fired! Out with him, by all means! There mustn't be a sign of the fellow here tomorrow!" Then he and the doctor would have dinner, and after dinner he would stretch out on his back on this raspberry-colored couch, cover his face with a newspaper and begin to snore after a good sleep he would have tea, and then drive the doctor over to his own place for the night. And the upshot of it all would be that the *feldscher* would remain in the hospital and the doctor would not resign.

But at heart the doctor wanted an altogether different denouement. His wish was that the *feldscher's* old aunt should be triumphant, that the board, in spite of his eight years of continuous service, should accept his resignation without a word of protest and, indeed, even with pleasure. He dreamed of how he would leave the hospital, to which he had got accustomed, how he would write a letter to the editor of *The Physician,* how his colleagues would tender him an address of sympathy. . . .

The siren appeared on the road. With a mincing gait and a swish of her dress, she walked over to the window and said:

"Grigory Ivanovich, will you be receiving the patients yourself or do you want us to receive them without you?"

Her eyes were saying: "You lost your temper, but now you have calmed down and you're ashamed of yourself; I am magnanimous, however, and don't notice it."

"I'll come right way," said the doctor.

He put on his apron, belted it with the towel, and went to the hospital.

"It wasn't right that I ran out after I struck him," he thought on the way. "It looked as though I were abashed or frightened. . . . I acted like a schoolboy. . . . It was all wrong!"

It seemed to him that when he entered the ward, the patients would look at him with embarrassment and that he, too, would be discomfited. But when he entered, the patients lay quietly in their beds and scarcely paid any attention to him. The face of the consumptive Gerasim expressed complete indifference and seemed to say: "You were put out with him and you have given him a dressing down. That's as it should be, brother."

The doctor opened two abscesses on the arm and bandaged it. Then he went to the women's ward, where he performed an operation on a peasant woman's eye. The siren was continually at his side and assisted him as though nothing had happened and everything were all right. Then came the turn of the ambulatory patients. In the doctor's small examining room the window was wide open. If you sat down on the windowsill and leaned over slightly, you could see the young grass two or three feet below. There had been a heavy thunderstorm the previous evening, and the grass looked somewhat trampled and glossy. The path which ran just beyond the window and led to the ravine looked washed clean, and the pieces of broken medicine bottles and jars scattered on both sides of it also looked washed, sparkling in the sun and sending out dazzling beams. Farther on, beyond the path, young firs garmented in luxuriant green, pressed close to one another; behind them loomed birches, their trunks white as paper, and through the foliage of the birches that trembled slightly in the breeze, you could see the blue, bottomless sky. When you looked out of the window, there were starlings hopping on the path, turning their foolish beaks in the direction of the window and debating with themselves: to get scared or not? Deciding to get scared, one by one they darted toward the treetops with a gay chirp, as if poking fun at the doctor who didn't know how to fly. . . .

The heavy smell of iodoform could not drown out the freshness and fragrance of the spring day. It was good to breathe!

"Anna Spiridonova!" the doctor called.

A young peasant woman in a red dress entered the examining room and turned to the icon, murmuring a prayer.

"What hurts you?" asked the doctor.

The woman glanced distrustfully at the door through which she had just entered and at the other door which led to the drug dispensary, came closer to the doctor, and whispered:

"No children!"

"Who hasn't registered yet?" the siren shouted from the dispensary. "Report here."

"He is a beast," the doctor thought to himself as he examined the patient, "just because he made me strike him. I never in my life struck anyone before."

Anna Spiridonova left. Next came an old man who had a venereal disease, then a peasant woman with three children, all suffering from scabies, and things began to hum. There was no sign of the *feldscher*. Behind the door in the drug dispensary the siren was making gay little noises, swishing her dress and clinking the bottles. Now and then she came into the examining room, to help with an operation or to fetch a prescription, and all with an air as though everything were as it should be.

"She's glad that I struck him," reflected the doctor, listening to the midwife's voice. "She and the *feldscher* were like cat and dog, and it will be a red letter day for her if he's discharged. I think the nurses are glad, too. . . . How disgusting!"

When he was at his busiest, he began to feel as though the midwife and the nurses, and the very patients, had purposely assumed an indifferent and even a cheerful expression. It was as though they understood that he was ashamed and pained, but out of delicacy they pretended not to. And he, wishing to show them that he was not ashamed, shouted roughly:

"Hey, you there! Shut the door, it's drafty!"

But he was ashamed and ill at ease. Having examined forty-five patients, he took his time leaving the hospital.

The midwife had already been to her quarters. A crimson kerchief round her shoulders, a cigarette between her teeth and a flower in her loose hair, she was hurrying off, either on a case or to visit friends. Patients sat on the porch and warmed themselves in the sun. The starlings were still making a racket and chasing beetles. The doctor looked about and reflected that among these untroubled existences of even tenor only two lives, his and the *feldscher's,* stuck out and were worthless, like two damaged piano keys. The *feldscher* must surely have gone to bed to sleep it off, but was probably unable to fall asleep because he knew that he was in a bad way, that he had been insulted and had lost his job. His position was excruciating. As for the doctor, who had never struck anyone, he felt as though he had lost his chastity. He no longer blamed the feldscher and exonerated himself, he was only perplexed: how had it happened that he, a decent fellow who had never struck even a dog, could have hit a man? Once in his lodging, he went to his study and lay down on the couch with his face to the back of it, and reflected thus:

"He's a wicked man, he does the patients no good; he's been with me three years now and I'm just fed up; still, what I did was inexcusable. I took advantage of the fact that I was the stronger of the two. He is my subordinate, he was at fault, and besides, he was drunk; I'm his superior, I was in the right and I was sober. And so I was the stronger. In the second place, I struck him in front of people who look up to me, and so I set them an abominable example."

The doctor was called to dinner. He had scarcely tasted the soup when he left the table and went to lie down again.

"What should I do then?" he continued communing with himself. "As soon as possible he must be given satisfaction. But how? As a hard-headed man, he probably thinks that a duel is stupid, or it doesn't mean anything to him. If I were to apologize to him in that very ward in front of the nurses and the patients, the apology would satisfy me but not him; being a horrid fellow, he would interpret my apology as cowardice, as fear that he would lodge a complaint against me with the authorities. Besides, the apology would just be the end of discipline in the hospital. Shall I offer him money? No, that is immoral and smacks of bribery. Or shall I put the problem up to our immediate superiors, that is, to the board? They could reprimand me or discharge me. But they won't. Besides, it's awkward to get the board mixed up in the intimate affairs of the hospital, and anyway the board has no legal right to deal with these things."

About three hours after dinner the doctor went down to the pond for a swim, and as he walked he was thinking to himself:

"And shouldn't I do what everyone does under such circumstances? Let him sue me. I am unquestionably guilty, I'll put up no defense, and the judge will send me to jail. In this way the injured party will receive satisfaction, and those who look up to me will see that I was in the wrong."

The idea appealed to him. He was pleased, and decided that the problem was settled and that there could be no happier solution.

"Well, that's fine!" he thought, getting into the water and watching the shoals of small golden crucians that were scurrying away from him. "Let him sue me. That will be all the easier for him because he's no longer on the job, and after this scandal one of us obviously must leave the hospital."

In the evening the doctor ordered his gig, intending to drive over to the captain's to play vint. As he stood in his study, in his coat and hat, putting on his gloves and ready to leave, the outer door opened creakingly and someone noiselessly entered the anteroom.

"Who's there?" the doctor called out.

"It's me, sir. . . ." a muffled voice answered.

The doctor felt his heart begin to pound and he was chilled through with shame and a kind of incomprehensible fear. Mikhail Zakharych (it was he) coughed softly, and timidly entered the study. After a pause, he said in a muffled, guilty tone of voice:

"Forgive me, Grigory Ivanovich!"

The doctor was taken aback and didn't know what to say. He realized that the *feldscher* had come to abase himself and apologize, not out of Christian humility, nor in order to heap coals of fire on the man who had insulted him, but simply for a sordid reason: "I'll force myself to apologize, and perhaps they won't fire me and take the bread out of my mouth. . . ." What could be more degrading?

"Forgive me. . . ." repeated the *feldscher*.

"Listen," began the doctor, without looking at him, and still not knowing what to say. "Listen. I insulted you and . . . I must suffer for it, that is, I must give you satisfaction. You're not the man to fight a duel. Nor am I, for that matter. I insulted you and you can lodge a complaint against me with the justice of the peace, and I'll take my punishment. But the two of us can't stay in the same place. One of us, you or I, must go! ('My God! I'm saying just the wrong thing!!' the doctor was horrified. 'How stupid, how stupid!') In a word, sue me! But we can't go on working together! It's either you or I! Lodge your complaint tomorrow!"

The *feldscher* looked at the doctor with a frown, and the frankest contempt flared up in his dark, turbid eyes. He had always thought the doctor was an impractical, capricious, puerile fellow, and now he despised him for his nervousness, for his incomprehensible, jerky way of speaking.

"I will bring suit," he said, with a look of sullen hatred.

"Well, do!"

"You think I won't sue you? I won't? I will. You've no right to use your fists on me. You ought to be ashamed of yourself! Only drunken peasants fight, and you're an educated man."

Suddenly the doctor's chest tightened with hatred, and in a voice that did not sound like his own he shouted:

"Get out!"

The *feldscher* reluctantly took a step or two (he looked as though he wanted to say something further), then walked into the anteroom and stood there, thinking. Having apparently made up his mind, he resolutely went out.

"How stupid, how stupid!" the doctor muttered, when the *feldscher* was gone. "How stupid and vulgar all this is!"

He felt that his behavior toward the man had been puerile, and he already realized that all his notions about the lawsuit were foolish, that they did not solve the problem but only complicated it.

"How stupid!" he repeated to himself, as he sat in his gig and later while he was playing vint at the captain's. "Is it possible that I am so badly educated and know life so little that I can't solve this simple problem? What shall I do?"

The next morning the doctor saw the *feldscher's* wife step into a carriage and reflected: "She must be going to his aunt's. Let her!"

The hospital managed to get along without a *feldscher*. It was necessary to notify the board, but the doctor was still unable to decide what form his letter should take. Now, it seemed to him, the tenor of the letter should be: "I request you to discharge the *feldscher,* although I am to blame, not he." For a decent person it was almost impossible to make this statement in a way which would not be stupid and shameful.

Two or three days later the doctor was informed that the *feldscher* had complained to Lev Trofimovich. The chairman hadn't let him say a word, had stamped his feet and chased him out, shouting: "I know you! Get out! I won't listen to you!" From there the *feldscher* had gone to the office of the Zemstvo and filed a report, in which he did not mention the slap in the face and asked nothing for himself, but informed the board that in his presence the doctor had several times commented unfavorably on the board and its chairman, that he treated patients in a manner contrary to accepted rules, that he was neglectful about making the prescribed rounds of his district, etc., etc. On learning of this, the doctor laughed, and thought: "What a fool!" And he felt shame and pity for the man who was behaving so foolishly; the more stupid things a man does in his defense, the weaker and more helpless he obviously is.

Exactly a week later the doctor received a summons from the justice of the peace.

"This is altogether absurd," he thought as he signed the necessary paper. "You couldn't conceive anything stupider."

As he was on his way to the court on a windless morning under an overcast sky, what he felt was not shame, but annoyance and disgust. He was vexed with himself, with the *feldscher,* with the situation.

"I'll up and say in court: 'To the devil with the lot of you!' " he raged inwardly. "You're all asses and you understand nothing!"

When he reached the building in which court was to be held, he saw in the doorway three of his nurses who had been called as witnesses, and the siren as well. In her impatience she was shifting her weight from one foot to the other, and she even blushed with pleasure when she beheld the principal character in the impending trial. The doctor, furious, was about to swoop down on them like a hawk and stun them by saying: "Who permitted you to leave the hospital? Be good enough to get back to your posts right away!" But he controlled himself and, pretending calmness, made his way through the crowd of peasants to the courtroom. The chamber was empty, and the justice's chain hung on the back of his armchair. The doctor went into the clerk's cubbyhole. There he saw a thin-faced young man wearing a cotton jacket with bulging pockets—it was the clerk—and the *feldscher.* He was sitting at a desk and, having nothing better to do, was paging a law journal. At the doctor's entrance the clerk rose, the *feldscher* looked abashed and rose also.

"Alexander Arkhipovich isn't here yet?" asked the doctor, embarrassed.

"Not yet, sir. He's in his own apartments," the clerk answered.

The court was located on the justice's estate, in one of the wings of his large house. The doctor left the court and walked unhurriedly toward the justice's apartments. He found Alexander Arkhipovich in the dining room, where a samovar was steaming. The justice, with his coat off and not even a waistcoat, his shirt open, so that his chest was bare, was standing at the table and, holding the tea-kettle with both hands, was pouring himself a tumbler of tea black as coffee. When he saw his visitor, he quietly drew another tumbler toward himself, filled it, and, without greeting the doctor, asked:

"With or without sugar?"

Long ago the justice of the peace had been in the cavalry, but now because for many years he had held elective offices he had the rank of Actual Councilor of State. Yet he had not discarded his army uniform or his military habits. He had long moustaches, the kind fancied by chiefs of police, wore trousers with piping, and all his gestures and words breathed military grace. He spoke with his head slightly thrown back, and garnishing his speech with the juicy, dignified "m'yeses" of a general, he swayed his shoulders and rolled his eyes. When he greeted you or gave you a light, he scraped his feet, and when he walked, he clinked his spurs as gently and cautiously as if every sound they made caused him intolerable pain. Having seated the doctor at table and provided him with tea, he stroked his broad chest and his stomach, heaved a deep sigh, and said:

"M'yes . . . Would you perhaps have some vodka and a bit to eat . . . m'yes?"

"No, thank you, I'm not hungry."

Both felt that they could not avoid the subject of the scandal at the hospital, and both felt awkward. The doctor was silent. The justice, with a graceful movement of the hand, caught an insect which had bit him on his chest, examined it carefully and let it go. Then he drew a deep sigh, looked up at the doctor, and, speaking deliberately, asked:

"Listen, why don't you send him packing?"

The doctor caught a note of sympathy in his voice; he was suddenly sorry for himself, and he felt tired and jaded by the disagreeable experiences he had endured in the course of the preceding week. His face showed that he had finally reached the end of his patience. He rose from the table, frowning irritably and shrugging his shoulders, and said:

"Send him packing! Good Lord, the logic of you people! It's astonishing, your logic! Don't you know that I can't send him packing? You sit here and think that I'm boss at the hospital and can do what I please! It's astonishing, your logic! Can I send the *feldscher* packing, if his aunt is employed as a nursemaid by Lev Trofimovich, and if Lev Trofimovich wants such gossip and flunkies as this Zakharych? What can I do if the Zemstvo people wipe the floor with us physicians, if they hinder us at every step? To hell with them, I don't want to work for them, that's all! I don't want to!"

"Well, well, well, old man. . . . You're making a mountain out of a molehill, you know. . . ."

"The marshal of the nobility goes out of his way to prove that we're all nihilists, he spies on us and treats us as his clerks. What right has he to come to the hospital in my absence and question the nurses and patients? Isn't it insulting? And this crazy Semyon Alexeich of yours, who does his own plowing and doesn't believe in medicine because he is as strong as an ox and eats like one, calls us parasites out loud and to our faces and begrudges us our salaries. Devil take him! I work day and night, I get no rest, I'm needed here more than all these psycho-paths, bigots, reformers, and all the other clowns taken together! I've made my-self sick with work, and what I get instead of gratitude is to have my salary thrown in my teeth! Many thanks! And everybody thinks he's entitled to stick his nose into what's none of his business, to teach me, to discipline me! At one meeting this Kamchatsky, a member of your board, reprimanded the physicians for wast-ing potassium iodide, and advised us to be careful in using cocaine! What does he know about it, I ask you? How's he concerned? Why doesn't he teach you how to run your court?"

"But he's a cad, my dear fellow, he's a bounder. . . . You mustn't pay any atten-tion to him. . . ."

"A cad, a bounder, and yet you've elected this character to the board and you allow him to stick his nose everywhere! You smile! According to you, these are trifles, bagatelles, but get it into your head that there are so many of these trifles that they make up my whole life, the way grains of sand make a mountain! I can't stand it any longer! I haven't the strength, Alexander Arkhipovich! A little more, and I'll not only use my fists on people, I'll draw a gun on them! Get into your head, my nerves aren't made of iron. I'm a human being like you. . . ."

Tears came to the doctor's eyes, and his voice quavered; he turned aside and looked out of the window. Silence fell.

"M'yes, my dear fellow. . . ." mumbled the justice thoughtfully. "On the other hand, to take a cold-blooded view . . ." (the justice caught a mosquito and, screw-ing his eyes tight, examined it carefully, crushed it and threw it into the slop-basin). "You see, there's no reason why he should be sent packing. Send him packing, and he'll be replaced by someone just like him or worse. You can try out a hun-dred men, and you won't find one you want to keep. . . . They're all no good." The justice stroked his armpits and then slowly lit a cigarette. "We must put up with it, bad as it is. Let me tell you that right now honest, sober, reliable workers can be found only among the intellectuals and the peasants, that is at the poles of society and only there. You can find a thoroughly honest physician, let's say, an excellent teacher, an honest plowman or a blacksmith, but the people in between, so to speak, those who no longer belong to the masses and who haven't yet be-come part of the intelligentsia, are an unreliable element. It's very hard to find an honest and sober *feldscher,* a clerk, a salesman, and so forth. Exceedingly hard! I've been in the courts since God knows when, and in all those years I've never had an honest, sober clerk, although I've tried out no end of them in my time. They are people who have no discipline, let alone principles, so to speak. . . ."

"Why is he talking this way?" thought the doctor. "Neither of us is saying what ought to be said."

"Here is a trick my own clerk played on me only last Friday," the justice continued. "In the evening he got together with some drunks, the devil knows who,
and all night long they were boozing in my chambers. How do you like that? I've
nothing against drinking. Devil take you, drink, but why bring utter strangers
into my chambers? Judge yourself: how long would it take to steal some document, say, a promissory note, from the files? And what do you think? After that
orgy I spent two days checking up to see if anything was missing. . . . Well, what
are you going to do about this wretch? Send him packing? Very well. . . . And what's
the guarantee that the next one won't be worse?"

"Besides, how can you send a man packing?" asked the doctor. "It's easy to say
it. How can I fire him and take the bread out of his mouth, when I know that he
is a family man and has nothing? Where would he go with his family?"

"Devil take it, I'm saying the wrong thing!" he thought to himself, and it seemed
odd to him that he could not fix his mind on some one definite idea or senti-
ment. "It's because I'm shallow and don't know how to think," he reflected.

"The man in-between, as you called him, is unreliable," he went on. "We send
him packing, scold him, slap him in the face, but we also ought to enter into his
situation. He is neither a peasant nor a master, neither fish, flesh, nor fowl. His
past is bleak, at present he has twenty-five rubles a month, a hungry family and a
job in which he's not his own master. The future holds the same twenty-five rubles
and the same dependent position, even if he holds on to his job for a hundred
years. He has neither education nor property; he has no time to go to church; he
doesn't profit by our example, because we don't let him get close enough to us.
So he goes on living like that, day in, day out, till he dies, without hoping for anything better, underfed, always afraid that any day he may be evicted from the quarters the Government provides him with, and that his children won't have a roof
over their heads. Under such circumstances, how is a man to keep from drinking,
from stealing? Under such conditions, how can he have principles?"

"So here we are, solving social problems!" the doctor thought to himself. "And
my God, how awkwardly! And what's all this for?"

The sound of bells was heard. Someone drove into the yard and halted before
the wing in which the court chambers were located and then went on and stopped
at the porch of the big house.

"Himself is here," said the justice, glancing out of the window. "Well, you'll get
it in the neck!"

"Please, let's be done with it, and fast," the doctor pleaded. "If possible, take
my case out of turn. I've no time, by Jove!"

"All right, all right. . . . Only, I don't know, old man, if the case is within my
jurisdiction. Your relations with the assistant were, so to speak, official, and, be-

sides, you smacked him while he was on duty. But I don't know for certain. Let's ask Lev Trofimovich."

Hurried steps were heard, and heavy breathing, and Lev Trofimovich, chairman of the board, a white-haired, bald-headed old man with a long beard and red eyelids, appeared in the doorway.

"Greetings!" he brought out, panting.

"Ouf! My dears! Tell them to bring me some kvass, judge! I can't stand it. . . ."

He sank into an armchair, but immediately jumped up, trotted over to the doctor and, staring at him angrily, said in a squeaking tenor:

"Many, many thanks to you, Grigory Ivanovich! You've done me a great favor, thank you! I won't forget it to my dying day, amen! Friends don't act like that! Say what you will, it's not decent of you. Why didn't you let me know? What do you think I am? Whom do you take me for? Am I your enemy or an utter stranger to you? Am I your enemy? Have I ever refused you anything? Eh?"

Staring hard and twiddling his fingers, the chairman drank kvass, wiped his lips hurriedly, and continued:

"Thank you very, very kindly! Why didn't you let me know? If you had any feeling for me, you would have driven up and talked to me as a friend: 'Lev Trofimovich, my dear fellow, the facts are so-and-so . . . This is what happened, and so on and so forth. . . .' Before you could turn round, I would have arranged everything, and there would have been no scandal . . . That fool has gone completely crazy, he wanders through the district, concocts stories and gossips with the women, and you, it's really shameful, if you'll excuse my saying so, you've started the devil knows what kind of a row, you've got that fool to sue you! It's shameful! Just shameful! Everybody asks me: What's the matter? What happened? How did it happen? And I, the chairman, know nothing of what's going on. You have no need of me! Many, many thanks, Grigory Ivanovich!"

The chairman made him such a low bow that he turned crimson, then he went over to the window and called:

"Zhigalov, ask Mikhail Zakharych to come here! Tell him to come up at once! It isn't right, my dear sir!" he said, walking away from the window. "Even my wife has taken offense, and you know how much she likes you. The trouble with you, gentlemen, is that you rely too much on reason! Everything has to be logical with you, you drag in principles, and worry about all the fine points, and as a result all you do is get things balled up!"

"And with you everything has to be illogical, and what is the result?" asked the doctor.

"What's the result? The result is that if I hadn't come here just now, you'd have disgraced yourself, and us, too. . . . It's just your luck that I came!"

The *feldscher* entered and stopped on the threshold. The chairman took up such a position that he was half turned away from the *feldscher,* put his hands in his pockets, cleared his throat, and said:

"Apologize to the doctor at once!"

The doctor flushed and ran into another room.

"You see, the doctor doesn't want to accept your apology!" the chairman went on. "He wants you to show that you're sorry not in words, but in deeds. Do you give your word of honor that from now on you will follow his orders and lead a sober life?"

"I do," the assistant brought out sullenly, in a deep voice.

"Watch out, then! And Heaven help you, if you don't! I'll fire you before you can say knife. If anything happens, don't come begging for mercy . . . Now, go on home. . . ."

For the *feldscher,* who had already accepted his misfortune, such a turn of events was a breath-taking surprise. So much so that he grew pale with joy. He wanted to say something, put out his hand, but could not bring out a word, smiled stupidly and left.

"That's that!" said the chairman. "And there's no need for any trial."

He drew a sigh of relief, and with an air of having just accomplished something difficult and important, he looked closely at the samovar and the glasses, rubbed his hands, and said:

"Blessed are the peacemakers. . . . Pour out a glass for me, Sasha. But wait, have them bring me a bite. . . . And, well, some vodka."

"Gentleman, this is absurd!" said the doctor, as he entered the dining-room, still flushed, and wringing his hands. "This . . . this is a comedy! It's vile! I can't bear it! It's better to have twenty trials than to settle matters in this farcical fashion. No, I can't stand it!"

"What do you want, then?" the chairman snapped at him. "Shall we fire him? Very well, I'll fire him."

"No, not that. I don't know what I want, but to take such an attitude towards life, gentlemen . . . Oh, my God! It's torture!"

The doctor started to bustle about nervously, looking for his hat, and failing to find it, sank into an armchair, exhausted.

"It's vile!" he repeated.

"My dear fellow," the justice muttered, "to some extent I fail to understand you, so to speak. . . . You're the one who is at fault in this affair, aren't you? To go about at the end of the nineteenth century, biffing people on the jaw, that is, not quite . . . so to speak. . . . He's a scoundrel, bu-u-ut, you will agree, you acted heedlessly, too."

"Of course!" the chairman chimed in.

Vodka and hors d'oeuvres were served.

Before taking his leave the doctor emptied a glass of vodka and ate a radish. As he was returning to the hospital, a mist, such as veils the grass on autumn mornings was beclouding his thoughts.

"Can it be," he reflected, "that after all that was said and thought and suffered during the past week, the end should be something so absurd and vulgar? How stupid! How stupid!"

He was ashamed of having involved strangers in his personal problem, ashamed of the things he had said to these people, ashamed of having drunk vodka out of a habit of idle drinking and idle living, ashamed of his blunt, shallow mind.

Back in the hospital, he immediately started making the rounds of the wards. The *feldscher* followed him, stepping softly like a cat, and answering questions gently. The *feldscher,* the siren, the nurses, all pretended that nothing had occurred and that everything was as it should be. The doctor himself made every effort to appear indifferent. He issued orders, fumed, cracked jokes with the patients, but in his brain a thought kept stirring:

"Stupid, stupid, stupid. . . ."

The Princess

A carriage with four fine sleek horses drove in at the big so-called Red Gate of the N—— Monastery. While it was still at a distance, the priests and monks who were standing in a group round the part of the hostel allotted to the gentry, recognized by the coachman and horses that the lady in the carriage was Princess Vera Gavrilovna, whom they knew very well.

An old man in livery jumped off the box and helped the princess to get out of the carriage. She raised her dark veil and moved in a leisurely way up to the priests to receive their blessing; then she nodded pleasantly to the rest of the monks and went into the hostel.

"Well, have you missed your princess?" she said to the monk who brought in her things. "It's a whole month since I've been to see you. But here I am; behold your princess. And where is the Father Superior? My goodness, I am burning with impatience! Wonderful, wonderful old man! You must be proud of having such a Superior."

When the Father Superior came in, the princess uttered a shriek of delight, crossed her arms over her bosom, and went up to receive his blessing.

"No, no, let me kiss your hand," she said snatching it and eagerly kissing it three times. "How glad I am to see you at last, holy Father! I'm sure you've forgotten your princess, but my thoughts have been in your dear monastery every moment. How delightful it is here! This living for God far from the busy, giddy world has a special charm of its own, holy Father, which I feel with my whole soul although I cannot express it!"

The princess's cheeks glowed and tears came into her eyes. She talked incessantly, fervently, while the Father Superior, a grave plain, shy man of seventy, remained mute or uttered abruptly, like a soldier on duty, phrases such as:

"Certainly, Your Excellency. . . . Quite so. I understand."

"Has Your Excellency come for a long stay?" he inquired.

"I shall stay the night here, and tomorrow I'm going on to Klavida Niko-laevna's—it's a long time since I've seen her—and the day after tomorrow I'll come back to you and stay three or four days. I want to rest my soul here among you, holy Father. . . ."

The princess liked being at the monastery at N——. For the last two years it had been a favorite resort of hers; she used to go there almost every month in the summer and stay two or three days, even sometimes a week. The shy novices, the stillness, the low ceilings, the smell of cypress, the modest fare, the cheap curtains on the windows—all this touched her, softened her, and disposed her to contemplation and good thoughts. It was enough for her to be half an hour in the hostel for her to feel that she, too, was timid and modest, and that she, too, smelt of cypress-wood. The past retreated into the background, lost its significance, and the princess began to imagine that in spite of her twenty-nine years she was very much like the old Father Superior, and that, like him, she was created not for wealth, not for earthly grandeur and love, but for a peaceful life secluded from the world, a life in twilight like the hostel.

It happens that a ray of light gleams in the dark cell of the anchorite absorbed in prayer, or a bird alights on the window and sings its song; the stern anchorite will smile in spite of himself, and a gentle, sinless joy will pierce through the load of grief over his sins, like water flowing from under a stone. The princess fancied she brought from the outside world just such comfort as the ray of light or the bird. Her gay, friendly smile, her gentle eyes, her voice, her jests, her whole personality in fact, her little graceful figure always dressed in simple black must arouse in simple, austere people a feeling of tenderness and joy. Everyone looking at her, must think: "God has sent us an angel. . . ." And feeling that no one could help thinking this, she smiled still more cordially, and tried to look like a bird.

After drinking tea and resting, she went for a walk. The sun was already setting. From the monastery garden came a moist fragrance of freshly watered mignonette, and from the church floated the soft singing of men's voices, which seemed very pleasant and mournful in the distance. It was the evening service. In the dark windows where the little lamps glowed gently, in the shadows, in the figure of the old monk sitting at the church door with a collecting-box, there was such unruffled peace that the princess felt moved to tears.

Outside the gate, in the walk between the wall and the birch trees where there were benches, it was a quiet evening. The air grew rapidly darker and darker. The princess went along the walk, sat on a seat, and sank into thought.

She thought how good it would be to settle down for her whole life in this monastery where life was as still and unruffled as a summer evening; how good it would be to forget the ungrateful, dissipated prince; to forget her immense estates, the creditors who worried her every day, her misfortunes, her maid Dasha, who had looked at her impertinently that morning. It would be nice to sit here on the bench all her life and watch through the trunks of the birch trees the evening mist gathering in wreaths in the valley below; the rooks flying home in a black cloud like a veil far, far away above the forest; two novices, one astride a piebald horse, another on foot driving out the horses for the night and rejoicing in their freedom, playing pranks like little children; their youthful voices rang out musically in the still air, and she could distinguish every word. It is nice to sit and listen to the silence: at one moment the wind blows and stirs the tops of the birch trees, then a frog rustles in last year's leaves, then the clock on the belfry strikes the quarter.... One might sit without moving, listen and think, and think....

An old woman passed by with a wallet on her back. The princess thought that it would be nice to stop the old woman and say something friendly and cordial to her, to help her.... But the old woman turned the corner without once looking round.

Not long afterwards a tall man with a gray beard and a straw hat came along the walk. When he came up to the princess, he took off his hat and bowed. From the bald patch on his head and his sharp, hooked nose the princess recognized him as the doctor, Mikhail Ivanovitch, who had been in her service at Dubovki. She remembered that someone had told her that his wife had died the year before, and she wanted to sympathize with him, to console him.

"Doctor, I expect you don't recognize me?" she said with an affable smile.

"Yes, Princess, I recognized you," said the doctor, taking off his hat again.

"Oh, thank you; I was afraid that you, too, had forgotten your princess. People only remember their enemies, but they forget their friends. Have you, too, come to pray?"

"I am the doctor here, and I have to spend the night at the monastery every Saturday."

"Well, how are you?" said the princess, sighing. "I hear that you have lost your wife. What a calamity!"

"Yes, Princess, for me it is a great calamity."

"There's nothing for it! We must bear our troubles with resignation. Not one hair of a man's head is lost without the Divine Will."

"Yes, Princess."

To the princess's friendly, gentle smile and her sighs the doctor responded coldly and dryly: "Yes Princess." And the expression of his face was cold and dry.

"What else can I say to him?" she wondered.

"How long it is since we met!" she said. "Five years! How much water has flowed under the bridge, how many changes in that time; it quite frightens one to think of it! You know, I am married.... I am not a countess now, but a princess. And by now I am separated from my husband too."

"Yes, I heard so."

"God has sent me many trials. No doubt you have heard, too, that I am almost ruined. My Dubovki, Sofyino, and Kiryakovo have all been sold for my unhappy husband's debts. And I have only Baranovo and Mihaltsevo left. It's terrible to look back: how many changes and misfortunes of all kinds, how many mistakes!"

"Yes, Princess, many mistakes."

The princess was a little disconcerted. She knew her mistakes; they were all of such private character that no one but she could think or speak of them. She could not resist asking:

"What mistakes are you thinking about?"

"You referred to them, so you know them. . . ." answered the doctor, and he smiled. "Why talk about them!"

"No; tell me, doctor. I shall be very grateful to you. And please don't stand on ceremony with me. I love to hear the truth."

"I am not your judge, Princess."

"Not my judge! What a tone you take! You must know something about me. Tell me!"

"If you really wish it, very well. Only I regret to say I'm not clever at talking, and people can't always understand me."

The doctor thought a moment and began:

"A lot of mistakes; but the most important of them, in my opinion, was the general spirit that prevailed on all your estates. You see, I don't know how to express myself. I mean chiefly the lack of love, the aversion for people that was felt in absolutely everything. Your whole system of life was built upon that aversion. Aversion for the human voice, for faces, for heads, steps . . . in fact, for everything that makes up a human being. At all the doors and on the stairs there stand sleek, rude and lazy grooms in livery to prevent badly dressed persons from entering the house; in the hall there are chairs with high backs so that the footmen waiting there, during balls and receptions, may not soil the walls with their heads; in every room there are thick carpets that no human step may be heard; everyone who comes in is infallibly warned to speak as softly and as little as possible, and to say nothing that might have a disagreeable effect on the nerves or the imagination. And in your room you don't shake hands with any one or ask him to sit down—just as you didn't shake hands with me or ask me to sit down. . . ."

"By all means, if you like," said the princess, smiling and holding out her hand. "Really, to be cross about such trifles. . . ."

"But I am not cross," laughed the doctor, but at once he flushed, took off his hat, and waving it about, began hotly: "To be candid, I've long wanted an opportunity to tell you all I think. . . . That is, I want to tell you that you look upon the mass of mankind from the Napoleonic standpoint as food for the cannon. But Napoleon had at least some idea; you have nothing except aversion."

"I have an aversion for people?" smiled the princess, shrugging her shoulders in astonishment. "I have!"

"Yes, you! You want facts? By all means. In Mihaltsevo three former cooks of yours, who have gone blind in your kitchen from the heat of the stove, are living upon charity. All the health and strength and good looks that is found on your hundreds of thousands of acres is taken by you and your parasites for your grooms, your footmen, and your coachman. All these two-legged cattle are trained to be flunkeys, overeat themselves, grow coarse, lose the 'image and likeness,' in fact. . . . Young doctors, agricultural experts, teachers, intellectual workers generally—think of it!—are torn away from their honest work and forced for a crust of bread to take part in all sorts of mummeries, which make every decent man feel ashamed! Some young men cannot be in your service for three years without becoming hypocrites, toadies, sneaks. . . . Is that a good thing? Your Polish superintendents, those abject spies, all those Kazimers and Kaetans go hunting about on your hundreds of thousands of acres from morning to night, and to please you try to get three skins off one ox. Excuse me, I speak disconnectedly, but that doesn't matter. You don't look upon the simple people as human beings. And even the princes, counts, and bishops who used to come and see you, you looked upon simply as decorative figures, not as living beings. But the worst of all, the thing that most revolts me, is having a fortune of over a million and doing nothing for other people, nothing!"

The princess sat amazed, aghast, offended, not knowing what to say or how to behave. She had never before been spoken to in such a tone. The doctor's unpleasant, angry voice and his clumsy, faltering phrases made a harsh clattering noise in her ears and her head. Then she began to feel as though the gesticulating doctor was hitting her on the head with his hat.

"It's not true!" she articulated softly, in an imploring voice. "I've done a great deal of good for other people; you know it yourself!"

"Nonsense!" cried the doctor. "Can you possibly go on thinking of your philanthropic work as something genuine and useful, and not a mere mummery? It was a farce from beginning to end; it was playing at loving your neighbor, the most open farce which even children and stupid peasant women saw through! Take for instance your—what was it called?—house for homeless old women without relations, of which you made me something like a head doctor, and which you were the patroness. Mercy on us! What a charming institution it was! A house was built with parquet floors and a weathercock on the roof; a dozen women were collected from the villages and made to sleep under blankets and sheets of Dutch linen, and given toffee to eat."

The doctor gave a malignant chuckle into his hat, and went on speaking rapidly and stammering:

"It was a farce! The attendant kept the sheets and blankets under lock and key, for fear the old women should soil them. 'Let the old devil's pepper-pots sleep on the floor.' The old women did not dare to sit down on the beds, to put on their jackets, to walk over the polished floors. Everything was kept for show and hidden away from the old women as though they were thieves, and the old women were clothed and fed on the sly by other people's charity, and prayed to God night and day to be released from their prison and from the canting exhortations of the sleek rascals to whose care you committed them. And what did the managers do? It was simply charming! About twice a week there would be thirty-five thousand messages to say that the princess—that is, you—were coming to the home next day. That meant the next day I had to abandon my patients, dress up and be on parade. Very good; I arrive. The old women, in everything clean and new, are already drawn up in a row, waiting. Near them struts the old garrison rat—the superintendent with his mawkish, sneaking smile. The old women yawn and exchange glances, but are afraid to complain. We wait. The junior steward gallops up. Half an hour later the senior steward; then the superintendent of the accounts' office, then another, and then another of them . . . they keep arriving endlessly. They all have mysterious solemn faces. We wait and wait, shift from one leg to another, look at the clock—all this is in monumental silence because we all hate each other like poison. One hour passes, then a second, and then at last the carriage is seen in the distance, and . . . and . . ."

The doctor went off into a shrill laugh and brought out in a shrill voice:

"You get out of the carriage, and the old hags, at the word of command from the garrison rat begin chanting: 'The Glory of our Lord Zion the tongue of man cannot express. . . . ' A pretty scene, wasn't it?"

The doctor went off into a bass chuckle, and waved his hand as though to signify that he could not utter another word for laughing. He laughed heavily, harshly, with clenched teeth, as ill-natured people laugh; and from his voice, from his face, from his glittering, rather insolent eyes it could be seen that he had a profound contempt for the princess, for the home, and for the old women. There was nothing amusing or laughable in all that he described so clumsily and coarsely, but he laughed with satisfaction, even with delight.

"And the school?" he went on, panting from laughter. "Do you remember how you wanted to teach peasant children yourself? You must have taught them very well, for very soon the children all ran away, so that they had to be thrashed and bribed to come and be taught. And you remember how you wanted to feed with your own hands the infants whose mothers were working in the fields. You went about the village crying because the infants were not at your disposal, as the mothers would take them to the fields with them. Then the village foreman ordered the mothers by turns to leave their infants behind for your entertainment. A strange thing! They all ran away from your benevolence like mice from a cat! And why was it? It's very simple. Not because our people are ignorant and ungrateful, as you always explained it to yourself, but because in all your fads, if you'll excuse the word, there wasn't a ha'p'orth of love and kindness! There was nothing but the desire to amuse yourself with living puppets, nothing else. . . . A person who does not feel the difference between a human being and a lap-dog ought not to go in for philanthropy. I assure you, there's a great difference between human beings and lap-dogs!"

The princess's heart was beating dreadfully; there was a thudding in her ears, and she still felt as though the doctor were beating her on the head with his hat. The doctor talked quickly, excitedly, and uncouthly, stammering and gesticulating unnecessarily. All she grasped was that she was spoken to by a coarse, ill-bred, spiteful, and ungrateful man; but what he wanted of her and what he was talking about, she could not understand.

"Go way!" she said in a tearful voice, putting up her hands to protect her head from the doctor's hat; "go way!"

"And how you treat your servants!" the doctor went on, indignantly. "You treat them as the lowest scoundrels, and don't look upon them as human beings. For example, allow me to ask, why did you dismiss me? For ten years I worked for your father and afterwards for you, honestly, without vacations or holidays. I gained the love of all for more than seventy miles round, and suddenly one fine day I am informed that I am no longer wanted. What for? I've no idea to this day. I, a doctor of medicine, a gentleman by birth, a student of the Moscow University, father of a family—am such a petty, insignificant insect that you can kick me out without explaining the reason! Why stand on ceremony with me! I heard afterwards that my wife went without my knowledge three times to intercede with you for me!—you wouldn't receive her. I am told she cried in your hall. And I shall never forgive her for it, never!"

The doctor paused and clenched his teeth, making an intense effort to think of something more to say, very unpleasant and vindictive. He thought of something, and his cold, frowning face suddenly brightened.

"Take your attitude to this monastery!" he said with avidity. "You've never spared any one, and the holier the place, the more chance of its suffering from your loving-kindness and angelic sweetness. Why do you come here? What do you want with the monks here, allow me to ask you? What is Hecuba to you or you to Hecuba? It's another farce, another amusement for you, another sacrilege against human dignity, and nothing more. Why, you don't believe in the monks' God; you've a God of your own in your heart, whom you've evolved for yourself at spiritualist séances. You look with condescension upon the ritual of the Church; you don't go to mass or vespers; you sleep till midday. . . . Why do you come here? . . . You come with a God of your own into a monastery you have nothing to do with, and you imagine that the monks look upon it as a very great honor. To be sure they do! You'd better ask, by the way, what your visits cost the monastery. You were graciously pleased to arrive here this evening, and a messenger from your estate arrived on horseback the day before yesterday to warn them of your coming. They were the whole day yesterday getting the rooms ready and expecting you. This morning your advance-guard arrived—an insolent maid, who keeps running across the courtyard rustling her skirts, pestering them with questions, giving orders. . . . I can't endure it! The monks have been on the lookout all day, for if you were not met with due ceremony, there would be trouble! You'd complain to the bishop! 'The monks don't like me, your holiness; I don't know what I've done to displease them. It's true I'm a great sinner, but I'm so unhappy!' Already one monastery has been in hot water over you. The Father Superior is a busy, learned man; he hasn't a free moment, and you keep sending for him to come to your rooms. Not a trace of respect for age or for rank! If at least you were a bountiful giver to the monastery, one wouldn't resent it so much, but all this time the monks have not received a hundred rubles from you!"

Whenever people worried the princess, misunderstood her, or mortified her, and when she did not know what to say or do, she usually began to cry. And on this occasion, too, she ended by hiding her face in her hands and crying aloud in a thin treble like a child. The doctor suddenly stopped and looked at her. His face darkened and grew stern.

"Forgive me, Princess," he said in a hollow voice. "I've given way to a malicious feeling and forgotten myself. It was not right."

And coughing in an embarrassed way, he walked away quickly, without remembering to put his hat on.

Stars were already twinkling in the sky. The moon must have been rising on the further side of the monastery, for the sky was clear, soft, and transparent. Bats were flitting noiselessly along the white monastery wall.

The clock slowly struck three quarters, probably a quarter to nine. The princess got up and walked slowly to the gate. She felt wounded and was crying, and she felt that the trees and the stars and even the bats were pitying her, and that the clock struck musically only to express its sympathy with her. She cried and thought how nice it would be to go into a monastery for the rest of her life. On still summer evenings she would walk alone through the avenues, insulted, injured, misunderstood by people, and only God and the starry heavens would see the martyr's tears. The evening service was still going on in the church. The princess stopped and listened to the singing; how beautiful the singing sounded in the still darkness! How sweet to weep and suffer to the sound of that singing!

Going into her rooms, she looked at her tear-stained face in the glass and powdered it, then she sat down to supper. The monks knew that she liked pickled sturgeon, little mushrooms, Malaga and plain honey-cakes that left a taste of cypress in the mouth, and every time she came they gave her all these dishes. As she ate the mushrooms and drank the Malaga, the princess dreamed of how she would be finally ruined and deserted—how all her stewards, bailiffs, clerks, and maid-servants for whom she had done so much, would be false to her, and begin to say rude things; how people all the world over would set upon her, speak ill of her, jeer at her. She would renounce her title, would renounce society and luxury, and would go into a convent without one word of reproach to any one; she would pray for her enemies—and then they would all understand her and come to beg her forgiveness, but by that time it would be too late.

After supper she knelt down in the corner before the icon and read two chapters of the Gospel. Then her maid made her bed and she got into it. Stretching herself under the white quilt, she heaved a sweet, deep sigh, as one sighs after crying, closed her eyes, and began to fall asleep.

In the morning she waked up and glanced at her watch. It was half-past nine. On the carpet near the bed was a bright, narrow streak of sunlight from a ray which came in at the window and dimly lighted up the room. Flies were buzzing behind the black curtain at the window. "It's early," thought the princess, and she closed her eyes.

Stretching and lying snug in her bed, she recalled her meeting yesterday with the doctor and all the thoughts with which she had gone to sleep the night before: she remembered she was unhappy. Then she thought of her husband living in Petersburg, her stewards, doctors, neighbors, the officials of her acquaintance. . . . a long procession of familiar masculine faces passed before her imagination. She smiled and thought, if only these people could see into her heart and understand her, they would all be at her feet.

At a quarter past eleven she called her maid.

"Help me to dress, Dasha," she said languidly. "But go first and tell them to get out the horses. I must set off for Klavdia Nikolaevna's."

Going out to get into the carriage, she blinked at the glaring daylight and laughed with pleasure: it was a wonderfully full day! As she scanned from her half-closed eyes the monks who had gathered round the steps to see her off, she nodded graciously and said:

"Good-bye, my friends! Till the day after tomorrow."

It was an agreeable surprise to her that the doctor was with the monks by the steps. His face was pale and severe.

"Princess," he said with a guilty smile, taking off his hat, "I've been waiting here a long time to see you. Forgive me, for God's sake . . . I was carried away yesterday by an evil, vindictive feeling and I talked . . . nonsense. In short, I beg your pardon."

The princess smiled graciously, and held out her hand for him to kiss. He kissed it, turning red.

Trying to look like a bird, the princess fluttered into the carriage and nodded in all directions. There was a gay, warm, serene feeling in her heart, and she felt herself that her smile was particularly soft and friendly. As the carriage rolled towards the gates, and afterwards along the dusty road past huts and gardens, past long trains of wagons and strings of pilgrims on their way to the monastery, she still screwed up her eyes and smiled softly. She was thinking there was no higher bliss than to bring warmth, light, and joy wherever one went, to forgive injuries, to smile graciously on one's enemies. The peasants she passed bowed to her, the carriage rustled softly, clouds of dust rose from under the wheels and floated over the golden rye, and it seemed to the princess that her body was swaying not on carriage cushions but on clouds, and that she herself was like a light, transparent little cloud. . . .

"How happy I am!" she murmured, shutting her eyes. "How happy I am!"

A Nervous Breakdown

A medical student called Mayer, and a pupil of the Moscow School of Painting, Sculpture, and Architecture called Rybnikov, went one evening to see their friend Vassilyev, a law student, and suggested that he should go with them to S. Street. For a long time Vassilyev would not consent to go, but in the end he put on his greatcoat and went with them.

He knew nothing of fallen women except by hearsay and from books, and he had never in his life been in the houses in which they lived. He knew that there are immoral women who, under the pressure of fatal circumstances—environment, bad education, poverty, and so on—are forced to sell their honor for money. They know nothing of pure love, have no children, have no civil rights; their mothers and sisters weep over them as though they were dead, science treats of them as an evil, men address them with contemptuous familiarity. But in spite of all that, they do not lose the semblance and image of God. They all acknowledge their sin and hope for salvation. Of the means that lead to salvation they can avail themselves to the fullest extent. Society, it is true, will not forgive people their past, but in the sight of God, St. Mary of Egypt is no lower than the other saints. When it had happened to Vassilyev in the street to recognize a fallen woman as such, by her dress or her manners, or to see a picture of one in a comic paper, he always remembered a story he had once read: a young man, pure and self-sacrificing, loves a fallen woman and urges her to become his wife; she, considering herself unworthy of such happiness, takes poison.

Vassilyev lived in one of the side streets turning out of Tverskoy Boulevard. When he came out of the house with his two friends it was about eleven o'clock. The first snow had not long fallen, and all nature was under the spell of the fresh snow. There was the smell of snow in the air, the snow crunched softly under the feet; the earth, the roofs, the trees, the seats on the boulevard, everything was soft, white, young, and this made the houses look quite different from the day before; the street lamps burned more brightly, the air was more transparent, the carriages rumbled with a deeper note, and with the fresh, light, frosty air a feeling stirred in the soul akin to the white, youthful, feathery snow. "Against my will an unknown force," hummed the medical student in his agreeable tenor, "has led me to these mournful shores."

"Behold the mill . . ." the artist seconded him, "in ruins now. . . ."

"Behold the mill . . . in ruins now," the medical student repeated, raising his eyebrows and shaking his head mournfully.

He paused, rubbed his forehead, trying to remember the words, and then sang aloud, so well that passers-by looked around:

"Here in old days when I was free,

Love, free, unfettered, greeted me."

The three of them went into a restaurant and, without taking off their greatcoats, drank a couple of glasses of vodka each. Before drinking the second glass, Vassilyev noticed a bit of cork in his vodka, raised the glass to his eyes, and gazed into it for a long time, screwing up his shortsighted eyes. The medical student did not understand his expression and said:

"Come, why look at it? No philosophizing, please. Vodka is given us to be drunk, sturgeon to be eaten, women to be visited, snow to be walked upon. For one evening anyway live like a human being!"

"But I haven't said anything. . . ." said Vassilyev, laughing. "Am I refusing to?"

There was a warmth inside him from the vodka. He looked with softened feelings at his friends, admired them and envied them. In these strong, healthy, cheerful people how wonderfully balanced everything is, how finished and smooth is everything in their minds and souls! They sing, and have a passion for the theater, and draw, and talk a great deal, and drink, and they don't have headaches the day after; they are both poetical and debauched, both soft and hard; they can work, too, and be indignant, and laugh without reason, and talk nonsense; they are warm, honest, self-sacrificing, and as men are in no way inferior to himself, Vassilyev, who watched every step he took and every word he uttered, who was fastidious and cautious, and ready to raise every trifle to the level of a problem. And he longed for one evening to let himself loose from his own control. If vodka had to be drunk, he would drink it, though his head would be splitting next morning. If he were taken to the women he would go. He would laugh, play the fool, gaily respond to the passing advances of strangers in the street.

He went out of the restaurant laughing. He liked his friends—one in a crushed broad-brimmed hat, with an affectation of artistic untidiness; the other in a sealskin cap, a man not poor, though he affected to belong to the Bohemia of learning. He liked the snow, the pale street lamps, the sharp black tracks left in the first snow by the feet of the passersby. He liked the air, and especially that limpid, tender, naïve, as it were virginal tone, which can be seen in nature only twice in the year—when everything is covered with snow, and in spring on bright days and moonlight evenings when the ice breaks on the river.

> "Against my will an unknown force,
>   Has led me to these mournful shores,"

he hummed in an undertone.

And the tune for some reason haunted him and his friends all the way, and all three of them hummed it mechanically, not in time with one another.

Vassilyev's imagination was picturing how, in another ten minutes, he and his friends would knock at a door; how by little dark passages and dark rooms they would steal in to the women; how, taking advantage of the darkness, he would strike a match, would light up and see the face of a martyr and a guilty smile. The unknown, fair or dark, would certainly have her hair down and be wearing a white dressing-jacket; she would be panic-stricken by the light, would be fearfully confused, and would say: "For God's sake, what are you doing! Put it out!" It would all be dreadful, but interesting and new.

II

The friends turned out of Trubnoy Square into Gratchevka, and soon reached the side street which Vassilyev only knew by reputation. Seeing two rows of houses with brightly lighted windows and wide-open doors, and hearing gay strains of pianos and violins, sounds which floated out from every door and mingled in a strange chaos, as though an unseen orchestra were tuning up in the darkness above the roofs, Vassilyev was surprised and said:

"What a lot of houses!"

"That's nothing," said the medical student. "In London there are ten times as many. There are about a hundred thousand such women there."

The cabmen were sitting on their boxes as calmly and indifferently as in any other side street; the same passers-by were walking along the pavement as in other streets. No one was hurrying, no one was hiding his face in his coat collar, no one shook his head reproachfully . . . And in this indifference to the noisy chaos of pianos and violins, to the bright windows and wide-open doors, there was a feeling of something very open, insolent, reckless, and devil-may-care. Probably it was as gay and noisy at the slave-markets in their day, and people's faces and movements showed the same indifference.

"Let us begin from the beginning," said the artist.

The friends went into a narrow passage lighted by a lamp with a reflector. When they opened the door a man in a black coat, with an unshaven face like a flunkey's and sleepy-looking eyes, got up lazily from a yellow sofa in the hall. The place smelt like a laundry with an odor of vinegar in addition. A door from the hall led into a brightly lighted room. The medical student and the artist stopped at this door and, craning their necks, peeped into the room.

"Buona sera, signori, rigolleto-hugenotti-traviata!" began the artist, with a theatrical bow.

"Havana-tarakano-pistoleto!" said the medical student, pressing his cap to his breast and bowing low.

Vassilyev was standing behind them. He would have liked to make a theatrical bow and say something silly, too, but he only smiled, felt an awkwardness that was like shame, and waited impatiently for what would happen next.

A little fair girl of seventeen or eighteen, with short hair, in a short light-blue frock with a bunch of white ribbon on her bosom, appeared in the doorway.

"Why do you stand at the door?" she said. "Take off your coats and come into the drawing-room."

The medical student and the artist, still talking Italian, went into the drawing room. Vassilyev followed them irresolutely.

"Gentlemen, take off your coats!" the flunkey said sternly; "you can't go in like that."

In the drawing-room there was, besides the girl, another woman, very stout and tall, with a foreign face and bare arms. She was sitting near the piano, laying out a game of patience on her lap. She took no notice whatsoever of the visitors.

"Where are the other young ladies?" asked the medical student.

"They are having their tea," said the fair girl.

"Stepan," she called, "go and tell the young ladies some students have come!"

A third young lady came into the room. She was wearing a bright red dress with blue stripes. Her face was painted thickly and unskillfully, her brow was hidden under her hair, and there was an unblinking, frightened stare in her eyes. As she came in, she began at once singing some song in a coarse, powerful contralto. After her a fourth appeared, and after her a fifth.

In all this Vassilyev saw nothing new or interesting. It seemed to him that the room, the piano, the looking-glass in its cheap gilt frame, the bunch of white ribbon, the dress with the blue stripes, and the blank indifferent faces, he had seen before and more than once. Of the darkness, the silence, the secrecy, the guilty smile, of all that he had expected to meet here and had dreaded, he saw no trace.

Everything was ordinary, prosaic, and uninteresting. Only one thing faintly stirred his curiosity—the terrible, as it were intentionally designed, bad taste which was visible in the cornices, in the absurd pictures, in the dresses, in the bunch of ribbons. There was something characteristic and peculiar in this bad taste.

"How poor and stupid it all is!" thought Vassilyev. "What is there in all this trumpery I see now that can tempt a normal man and excite him to commit the horrible sin of buying a human being for a ruble? I understand any sin for the sake of splendor, beauty, grace, passion, taste; but what is there here? What is there here worth sinning for? But . . . one mustn't think!"

"Beardy, treat me to some porter!" said the fair girl, addressing him.

Vassilyev was at once overcome with confusion.

"With pleasure," he said, bowing politely. "Only excuse me, madam, I . . . I won't drink with you. I don't drink."

Five minutes later the friends went off into another house.

"Why did you ask for porter?" said the medical student angrily. "What a millionaire! You have thrown away six rubles for no reason whatever—simply waste!"

"If she wants it, why not let her have the pleasure?" said Vassilyev, justifying himself.

"You did not give pleasure to her, but to the 'Madame.' They are told to ask the visitors to stand them treat because it is a profit to the keeper."

"Behold the mill . . ." hummed the artist, "in ruins now . . ."

Going into the next house, the friends stopped in the hall and did not go to the drawing room. Here, as in the first house, a figure in a black coat, with a sleepy face like a flunkey's, got up from a sofa in the hall. Looking at this flunkey, at his face and his shabby black coat, Vassilyev thought: "What must an ordinary simple Russian have gone through before fate flung him down as a flunkey here? Where had he been before and what had he done? What was awaiting him? Was he married? Where was his mother, and did she know that he was a servant here?" And Vassilyev could not help particularly noticing the flunkey in each house. In one of the houses—he thought it was the fourth—there was a little spare, frail-looking flunkey with a watch-chain on his waistcoat. He was reading a newspaper, and took no notice of them when they went in. Looking in his face Vassilyev, for some reason, thought that a man with such a face might steal, might murder, and might bear false witness. But the face was really interesting: a big forehead, gray eyes, a little flattened nose, thin compressed lips, and a blankly stupid and at the same time insolent expression like that of a young harrier overtaking a hare. Vassilyev thought it would be nice to touch this man's hair, to see whether it was soft or coarse. It must be coarse like a dog's.

III

Having drunk two glasses of porter, the artist became suddenly tipsy and grew unnaturally lively.

"Let's go to another!" he said peremptorily, waving his hands. "I will take you to the best one."

When he had brought his friends to the house that in his opinion was the best, he declared his firm intention of dancing a quadrille. The medical student grumbled something about their having to pay the musicians a ruble, but agreed to be his *vis-à-vis*. They began dancing.

It was just as nasty in the best house as in the worst. Here there were just the same looking-glasses and pictures, the same styles of coiffure and dress. Looking round at the furnishing of the rooms and the costumes, Vassilyev realized that this was not lack of taste, but something that might be called the taste, and even the style, of S. Street, which could not be found elsewhere—something intentional in its ugliness, not accidental, but elaborated in the course of years. After he had been in eight houses, he was no longer surprised at the color of the dresses, at the long trains, the gaudy ribbons, the sailor dresses, and the thick purplish rouge on the cheeks; he saw that it all had to be like this, that if a single one of the women had been dressed like a human being, or if there had been one decent engraving on the wall, the general tone of the whole street would have suffered.

"How unskillfully they sell themselves!" he thought. "How can they fail to understand that vice is only alluring when it is beautiful and hidden, when it wears the mask of virtue? Modest black dresses, pale faces, mournful smiles, and darkness would be far more effective than this clumsy tawdriness. Stupid things! If they don't understand it of themselves, their visitors might surely have taught them. . . ."

A young lady in a Polish dress edged with white fur came up to him and sat down beside him.

"You nice dark man, why aren't you dancing?" she asked. "Why are you so dull?"

"Because it is dull."

"Treat me to some Lafitte. Then it won't be dull."

Vassilyev made no answer. He was silent for a little, and then asked:

"What time do you get to sleep?"

"At six o'clock."

"And what time do you get up?"

"Sometimes at two and sometimes at three."

"And what do you do when you get up?"

"We have coffee, and at six o'clock we have dinner."

"And what do you have for dinner?"

"Usually soup, beefsteak, and dessert. Our madam keeps the girls well. But why do you ask all this?"

"Oh, just to talk. . . . ."

Vassilyev longed to talk to the young lady about many things. He felt an intense desire to find out where she came from, whether her parents were living, and whether they knew that she was here; how she had come into this house; whether she were cheerful and satisfied, or sad and oppressed by gloomy thoughts; whether she hoped some day to get out of her present position. But he could not think how to begin or in what shape to put his questions so as not to seem impertinent. He thought for a long time, and asked:

"How old are you?"

"Eighty," the young lady jested, looking with a laugh at the antics of the artist as he danced.

All at once she burst out laughing at something, and uttered a long cynical sentence loud enough to be heard by everyone. Vassilyev was aghast, and not knowing how to look, gave a constrained smile. He was the only one who smiled; all the others, his friends, the musicians, the women, did not even glance towards his neighbor, but seemed not to have heard her.

"Stand me some Lafitte," his neighbor said again.

Vassilyev felt a repulsion for her white fur and for her voice, and walked away from her. It seemed to him hot and stifling, and his heart began throbbing slowly but violently, like a hammer—one! two! three!

"Let us go away!" he said, pulling the artist by his sleeve.

"Wait a little; let me finish."

While the artist and the medical student were finishing the quadrille, to avoid looking at the women, Vassilyev scrutinized the musicians. A respectable-looking old man in spectacles rather like Marshal Bazaine, was playing the piano; a young man with a fair beard, dressed in the latest fashion, was playing the violin. The young man had a face that did not look stupid nor exhausted, but intelligent, youthful, and fresh. He was dressed fancifully and with taste; he played with feeling. It was a mystery how he and the respectable-looking old man had come here. How was it they were not ashamed to sit here? What were they thinking about when they looked at the women?

If the violin and the piano had been played by men in rags, looking hungry, gloomy, drunken, with dissipated or stupid faces, then one could have understood their presence, perhaps. As it was, Vassilyev could not understand it all. He recalled the story of the fallen woman he had once read, and he thought now that that human figure with the guilty smile had nothing in common with what he was seeing now. It seemed to him that he was seeing not fallen women, but some different world quite apart, alien to him and incomprehensible; if he had seen this world before on the stage, or read of it in a book, he would not have believed in it.

The woman with the white fur burst out laughing again and uttered a loathsome sentence in a loud voice. A feeling of disgust took possession of him. He flushed crimson and went out of the room.

"Wait a minute, we are coming too!" the artist shouted to him.

IV

"While we were dancing," said the medical student, as they all three went out into the street, "I had a conversation with my partner. We talked about her first romance. He, the hero, was an accountant at Smolensk with a wife and five children. She was seventeen, and she lived with her papa and mamma, who sold soap and candles."

"How did he win her heart?" asked Vassilyev.

"By spending fifty rubles on underclothes for her. What next!"

"So he knew how to get his partner's story out of her," thought Vassilyev about the medical student. "But I don't know how to."

"I say, I am going home!" he said.

"What for?"

"Because I don't know how to behave here. Besides, I am bored, disgusted. What is there amusing in it? If they were human beings—but they are savages and animals. I am going; do as you like."

"Come, Grisha, Grigory, darling . . . " said the artist in a tearful voice, hugging Vassilyev, "come along! Let's go to one more together and damnation take them! Please do, Grisha!"

They persuaded Vassilyev and led him up a staircase. In the carpet and the gilt banisters, in the reporter who opened the door, and in the panels that decorated the hall, the same S. Street style was apparent, but carried to a greater perfection, more imposing.

"I really will go home!" said Vassilyev as he was taking off his coat.

"Come, come, dear boy," said the artist, and he kissed him on the neck. "Don't be tiresome. Gri-gri, be a good comrade! We came together, we will go back together. What a beast you are, really!"

"I can wait for you in the street. I think it's loathsome, really!"

"Come, come, Grisha. If it is loathsome, you can observe it! Do you understand? You can observe!"

"One must take an objective view of things," said the medical student gravely.

Vassilyev went into the drawing room and sat down. There were a number of visitors in the room besides him and his friends: two infantry officers, a bald, gray-haired gentleman in spectacles, two beardless youths from the institute of land-surveying, and a very tipsy man who looked like an actor. All the young ladies were taken up with these visitors and paid no attention to Vassilyev.

Only one of them, dressed *à la Aida,* glanced sideways at him, smiled and said yawning: "A dark one has come."

Vassilyev's heart was throbbing and his face burned. He felt ashamed before these visitors of his presence here, and he felt disgusted and miserable. He was tormented by the thought that he, a decent and loving man (such as he had hitherto considered himself), hated these women and felt nothing but repulsion towards them. He felt pity neither for the women nor the musicians nor the flunkeys.

"It is because I am not trying to understand them," he thought. "They are all more like animals than human beings, but of course they are human beings all the same, they have souls. One must understand them and then judge."

"Grisha, don't go, wait for us," the artist shouted to him and disappeared.

The medical student disappeared soon after.

"Yes, one must make an effort to understand, one mustn't be like this." Vassilyev went on thinking.

And he began gazing at each of the women with strained attention, looking for a guilty smile. But either he did not know how to read their faces, or not one of these women felt herself to be guilty; he read on every face nothing but a blank expression of everyday vulgar boredom and complacency. Stupid faces, stupid smiles, harsh, stupid voices, insolent movements, and nothing else. Apparently each of them had in the past a romance with an accountant based on underclothes for fifty rubles, and looked for no other charm in the present but coffee, a dinner of three courses, wines, quadrilles, sleeping till two in the afternoon. . . . .

Finding no guilty smile, Vassilyev began to look whether there was not one intelligent face. And his attention was caught by one pale, rather sleepy exhausted-looking face. It was a dark woman, not very young, wearing a dress covered with spangles; she was sitting in an easy chair, looking at the floor lost in thought. Vassilyev walked from one corner of the room to the other, and, as though casually, sat down beside her.

"I must begin with something trivial," he thought, "and pass to what is serious."

"What a pretty dress you have," and with his finger he touched the gold fringe of her fichu.

"Oh, is it?" said the dark woman listlessly.

"What province do you come from?"

"I? From a distance. . . . . From Tchernigov."

"A fine province. It's nice there."

"Any place seems nice when one is not in it."

"It's a pity I cannot describe nature," thought Vassilyev. "I might touch her by a description of nature in Tchernigov. No doubt she loves the place if she has been born there."

"Are you dull here?" he asked.

"Of course I am dull."

"Why don't you go away from here if you are dull?"

"Where should I go to? Go begging or what?"

"Begging would be easier than living here."

"How do you know that? Have you begged?"

"Yes, when I hadn't the money to study. Even if I hadn't anyone could understand that. A beggar is anyway a free man, and you are a slave."

The dark woman stretched, and watched with sleepy eyes the footman who was bringing a trayful of glasses and seltzer water.

"Stand me a glass of porter," she said, and yawned again.

"Porter," thought Vassilyev. "And what if your brother or mother walked in at this moment? What would you say? And what would they say? There would be porter then, I imagine."

All at once there was the sound of weeping. From the adjoining room, from which the footman had brought the seltzer water, a fair man with a red face and angry eyes ran in quickly. He was followed by the tall, stout "madam," who was shouting in a shrill voice:

"Nobody has given you leave to slap the girls on the cheeks! We have visitors better than you, and they don't fight! Imposter!"

A hubbub arose. Vassilyev was frightened and turned pale. In the next room there was the sound of bitter, genuine weeping, as though of someone insulted. And he realized that there were real people living here who, like people everywhere else, felt insulted, suffered, wept, and cried for help. The feeling of oppressive hate and disgust gave way to an acute feeling of pity and anger against the aggressor. He rushed in the room where there was weeping. Across rows of bottles on a marble-top table he distinguished a suffering face, wet with tears, stretched out his hands towards that face, took a step towards the table, but at once drew back in horror. The weeping girl was drunk.

As he made his way through the noisy crowd gathered about the fair man, his heart sank and he felt frightened like a child; and it seemed to him that in this alien, incomprehensible world people wanted to pursue him, to beat him, to pelt him with filthy words. He tore down his coat from the hat stand and ran headlong downstairs.

V

Leaning against the fence, he stood near the house waiting for his friends to come out. The sounds of the pianos and violins, gay, reckless, insolent, and mournful, mingled in the air in a sort of chaos, and this tangle of sounds seemed again like an unseen orchestra tuning up on the roofs. If one looked upwards into the darkness, the black background was all spangled with white, moving spots: it was snow falling. As the snowflakes came into the light they floated round lazily in the air like down, and still more lazily fell to the ground. The snowflakes whirled thickly round Vassilyev and hung upon his beard, his eyelashes, his eyebrows. The cabmen, the horses, and the passers-by were white.

"And how can the snow fall in this street!" thought Vassilyev. "Damnation takes these houses!"

His legs seemed to be giving way from fatigue, simply from having run down the stairs; he gasped for breath as though he had been climbing uphill, his heart beat so loudly that he could hear it. He was consumed by a desire to get out of the street as quickly as possible and to go home, but even stronger was his desire to wait for his companions and vent upon them his oppressive feeling.

There was much he did not understand in these houses, the souls of ruined women were a mystery to him as before; but it was clear to him that the thing was far worse than could have been believed. If that sinful woman who had poisoned herself was called fallen, it was difficult to find a fitting name for all these who were dancing now to this tangle of sound and uttering long, loathsome sentences. They were not on the road to ruin, but ruined.

"There is vice," he thought, "but neither consciousness of sin nor hope of salvation. They are sold and bought, steeped in wine and abominations, while they, like sheep, are stupid, indifferent, and don't understand. My God! My God!"

It was clear to him, too, that everything that is called human dignity, personal rights, the Divine image and semblance, were defiled to their very foundations— "to the very marrow," as drunkards say—and that not only the street and the stupid women were responsible for it.

A group of students, white with snow, passed him, laughing and talking gaily; one, a tall thin fellow, stopped, glanced into Vassilyev's face, and said in a drunken voice:

"One of us! A bit on, old man? Aha-ha! Never mind, have a good time! Don't be down-hearted, old chap!"

He took Vassilyev by the shoulder and pressed his cold wet mustache against his cheek, then he slipped, staggered, and, waving both hands, cried:

"Hold on! Don't upset!"

And laughing, he ran to overtake his companions.

Through the noise came the sound of the artist's voice:

"Don't you dare hit the women! I won't let you, damnation take you! You scoundrels!"

The medical student appeared in the doorway. He looked from side to side, and seeing Vassilyev, said in an agitated voice:

"You here! I tell you it's really impossible to go anywhere with Yegor! What a fellow he is! I don't understand him! He has got up a scene! Do you hear? Yegor!" he shouted at the door. "Yegor!"

"I won't allow you to hit women!" the artist's piercing voice sounded from above. Something heavy and lumbering rolled down the stairs. It was the artist falling headlong. Evidently he had been pushed downstairs.

He picked himself up from the ground, shook his hat, and with an angry and indignant face, brandished his fist towards the top of the stairs and shouted:

"Scoundrels! Torturers! Bloodsuckers! I won't allow you to hit them! To hit a weak, drunken woman! Oh, you brutes."

"Yegor! come, Yegor!" the medical student began imploring him. "I give you my word of honor I'll never come with you again. On my word of honor I won't!"

Little by little the artist was pacified and the friends went homewards.

"Against my will an unknown force," hummed the medical student, "had led me to these mournful shores."

"Behold the mill," the artist chimed in a little later, "in ruins now. What a lot of snow, Holy Mother! Grisha, why did you go? You are a funk, a regular old woman."

Vassilyev walked behind his companions, looked at their backs, and thought:

"One of two things: either we only fancy prostitution is an evil, and we exaggerate it; or, if prostitution really is as great an evil as is generally assumed, these dear friends of mine are as much slave-owners, violators, and murderers, as the inhabitants of Syria and Cairo, that are described in the 'Neva.' Now they are singing, laughing, talking sense, but haven't they just been exploiting hunger, ignorance, and stupidity? They have—I have been a witness of it. What is the use of their humanity, their medicine, their painting? The science, art, and lofty sentiments of these soul-destroyers remind me of the piece of bacon in the story. Two brigands murdered a beggar in a forest; they began sharing his clothes between them, and found in his wallet a piece of bacon. 'Well found,' said one of them; 'let us have a bit.' 'What do you mean? How can you?' cried the other in horror. 'Have you forgotten that today is Wednesday?' And they would not eat it. After murdering a man, they came out of the forest in the firm conviction that they were keeping the fast. In the same way these men, after buying women, go their way imagining that they are artists and men of science."

"Listen!" he said sharply and angrily. "Why do you come here? Is it possible—is it possible that you don't understand how horrible it is? Your medical books tell you that every one of these women dies prematurely of consumption or something; art tells you that morally they are dead even earlier. Every one of them dies because she has in her time to entertain five hundred men on an average, let us say. You are among those five hundred! If each of you in the course of your lives visits this place or others like it two hundred and fifty times, it follows that one woman is killed for every two of you! Can't you understand that? Isn't it horrible to murder, two of you, three of you, five of you, a foolish, hungry woman! Ah! Isn't it awful, my God!"

"I knew it would end like that," the artist said frowning. "We ought not to have gone with this fool and ass! You imagine you have grand notions in your head now, ideas, don't you? No, it's the devil knows what, but not ideas. You are looking at me now with hatred and repulsion, but I tell you it's better you should set up twenty more houses like those than look like that. There's more vice in your expression than in the whole street! Come along, Volodya, let him go to the devil! He's a fool and an ass, and that's all."

"We human beings do murder each other," said the medical student. "It's immoral, of course, but philosophizing doesn't help it. Good-by!"

At Trubnoy Square the friends said good-by and parted. When he was left alone, Vassilyev strode rapidly along the boulevard. He felt frightened of the darkness, of the snow which was falling in heavy flakes on the ground, and seemed as though it would cover up the whole world; he felt frightened of the street lamps shining with pale light through the clouds of snow. His soul was possessed by an unaccountable, faint-hearted terror. Passers-by came towards him from time to time, but he timidly moved to one side; it seemed to him that women, none but women, were coming from all sides and staring at him.

"It's beginning," he thought, "I am going to have a breakdown."

VI

At home he lay on his bed and said, shuddering all over; "They are alive! Alive! My God, those women are alive!"

He encouraged his imagination in all sorts of ways to picture himself the brother of a fallen woman, or her father; then a fallen woman herself, with her painted cheeks; and it all moved him to horror.

It seemed to him that he must settle the question at once at all costs, and that this question was not one that did not concern him, but was his own personal problem. He made an immense effort, repressed his despair, and sitting on the bed, holding his head in his hands, began thinking how one could save all the women he had seen that day. The method for attacking problems of all kinds was, as he was an educated man, well known to him. And however excited he was, he strictly adhered to that method. He recalled the history of the problem and its literature, and for a quarter of an hour he paced from one end of the room to the other trying to remember all the methods practiced at the present time for saving women. He had very many good friends and acquaintances who lived in lodgings in Petersburg. Among them were a good many honest and self-sacrificing men. Some of them had attempted to save women.

"All these not very numerous attempts," thought Vassilyev, "can be divided into three groups. Some, after buying the woman out of the brothel, took a room for her, bought her a sewing machine, and she became a seamstress. And whether he wanted to or not, after having bought her out he made her his mistress; then when he had taken his degree, he went away and handed her into the keeping of some other decent man as though she were a thing. And the fallen woman remained a fallen woman. Others, after buying her out, took a lodging apart for her, bought the inevitable sewing-machine, and tried teaching her to read, preaching at her and giving her books. The woman lived and sewed as long as it was interesting and a novelty to her, then getting bored, began receiving men on the sly, or ran away and went back where she could sleep till three o'clock, drink coffee, and have good dinners. The third class, the most ardent and self-sacrificing, had taken a bold, resolute step. They had married them. And when the insolent and spoilt, or stupid and crushed animal became a wife, the head of a household, and afterwards a mother, it turned her whole existence and attitude to life upside down, so that it was hard to recognize the fallen woman afterwards in the wife and the mother. Yes, marriage was the best and perhaps the only means."

"But it is impossible!" Vassilyev said aloud, and he sank upon his bed. "I, to begin with, could not marry one! To do that one must be a saint and be unable to feel hatred or repulsion. But supposing that I, the medical student, and the artist mastered ourselves and did marry them—suppose they were all married. What would be the result? The result would be that while here in Moscow they were being married, some Smolensk accountant would be debauching another lot, and that lot would be streaming here to fill the vacant places, together with the others from Saratov, Nizhni-Novgorod, Warsaw. And what is one to do with the hundred thousand in London? What's one to do with those in Hamburg?"

The lamp in which the oil had burnt down began to smoke. Vassilyev did not notice it. He began pacing to and fro again, still thinking. Now he put the questions differently: what must be done that fallen women should not be needed? For that, it was essential that the men who buy them and do them to death should feel all the immorality of their share in enslaving them and should be horrified. One must save the men.

"One won't do anything by art and science, that is clear," thought Vassilyev. "The only way out of it is missionary work."

And he began to dream how he would the next evening stand at the corner of the street and say to every passer-by: "Where are you going and what for? Have some fear of God!"

He would turn to the apathetic cabmen and say to them: "Why are you staying here? Why aren't you revolted? Why aren't you indignant? I suppose you believe in God and know that it is a sin, the people go to hell for it? Why don't you speak? It is true that they are strangers to you, but you know even they have fathers, brothers like yourselves."

One of Vassilyev's friends had once said of him that he was a talented man. There are all sorts of talents—talent for writing, talent for the stage, talent for art; but he had a peculiar talent—a talent for humanity. He possessed an extraordinarily fine delicate scent for pain in general. As a good actor reflects himself the movements and voice of others, so Vassilyev could reflect in his soul the sufferings of others. When he saw tears, he wept; beside a sick man, felt sick himself and moaned; if he saw an act of violence, he felt as though he himself were the victim of it, he was frightened as a child, and in his fright ran to help. The pain of others worked on his nerves, excited him, roused him to a state of frenzy, and so on.

Whether this friend was right I don't know, but what Vassilyev experienced when he thought this question was settled was something like inspiration. He cried and laughed, spoke aloud the words that he should say next day, felt a fervent love for those who would listen to him and would stand beside him at the corner of the street to preach; he sat down to write letters, and made vows to himself.

All this was like inspiration from the fact that it did not last long. Vassilyev was soon tired. The cases in London, in Hamburg, in Warsaw, weighed upon him by their mass as a mountain weighs upon the earth; he felt dispirited, bewildered, in the face of this mass; he remembered that he had not a gift for words, that he was cowardly and timid, that indifferent people would not be willing to listen and understand him, a law student in his third year, a timid and insignificant person; that genuine missionary work included not only teaching but deeds.

When it was daylight and carriages were already beginning to rumble in the street, Vassilyev was lying motionless on the sofa, staring into space. He was no longer thinking of the women, nor of the men, nor of missionary work. His whole attention was turned upon the spiritual agony which was torturing him. It was a dull, vague, undefined anguish akin to misery, to an extreme form of terror, and to despair. He could point to the place where the pain was, in his breast under his heart; but he could not compare it with anything. In the past he had had acute toothache, he had had pleurisy and neuralgia, but all that was insignificant compared with this spiritual anguish. In the presence of that pain life seemed loathsome. The dissertation, the excellent work he had written already, the people he loved, the salvation of fallen women—everything that only the day before he had cared about or been indifferent to, now when he thought of them irritated him in the same way as the noise of the carriages, the scurrying footsteps of the waiters in the passage, the daylight. If at that moment someone had performed a great deed of mercy or had committed a revolting outrage, he would have felt the same repulsion for both actions. Of all the thoughts that strayed through his mind only two did not irritate him: one was that at every moment he had the power to kill himself, the other that this agony would not last more than three days. This last he knew by experience.

After lying for a while he got up and, wringing his hands, walked about the room, not as usual from corner to corner, but round the room beside the walls. As he passed he glanced at himself in the looking glass. His face looked pale and sunken, his temples looked hollow, his eyes were bigger, darker, more staring, as though they belonged to someone else, and they had an expression of insufferable mental agony.

At midday the artist knocked at the door.

"Grigory, are you at home?" he asked.

Getting no answer, he stood for a minute, pondered, and answered himself in Little Russian: "Nay. The confounded fellow has gone to the University."

And he went away. Vassilyev lay down on the bed and, thrusting his head under the pillow, began crying with agony, and the more freely his tears flowed the more terrible his mental anguish became. As it began to get dark, he thought of the agonizing night awaiting him, and was overcome by a horrible despair. He dressed quickly, ran out of his room, and, leaving his door wide open, for no object or reason went out into the street. Without asking himself where he should go, he walked quickly along Sadovoy Street.

Snow was falling as heavily as the day before; it was thawing. Thrusting his hands into his sleeves, shuddering and frightened at the noises, at the tram bells, and at the passers-by, Vassilyev walked along Sadovoy Street as far as Suharev Tower; then to the Red Gate; from there he turned off to Basmannya Street. He went into a tavern and drank off a big glass of vodka, but that did not make him feel better. When he reached Razgulya he turned to the right, and strode along side streets in which he had never been before in his life. He reached the old bridge by which the Yauza runs gurgling, and from which one can see long rows of lights in the windows of the Red Barracks. To distract his spiritual anguish by some sensation or some other pain, Vassilyev, not knowing what to do, crying and shuddering, undid his greatcoat and jacket and exposed his bare chest to the wet snow and the wind. But that did not lessen his suffering either. Then he bent down over the rail of the bridge and looked down into the black, yeasty Yauza, and he longed to plunge down head-foremost; not from loathing for life, not for the sake of suicide, but in order to bruise himself at least, and by one pain to ease the other. But the black water, the darkness, the deserted banks covered with snow were terrifying. He shivered and walked on. He walked up and down by the Red Barracks, then turned back and went down to a copse, from the copse back to the bridge again.

"No, home, home!" he thought. "At home I believe it's better. . . ."

And he went back. When he reached home he pulled off his wet coat and cap, began pacing around the room, and went on pacing round and round without stopping till morning.

VII

When next morning the artist and the medical student went in to him, he was moving about the room with his shirt torn, biting his hands and moaning with pain.

"For God's sake!" he sobbed when he saw his friends, "take me where you please, do what you can; but for God's sake, save me quickly! I shall kill myself!"

The artist turned pale and was helpless. The medical student, too, almost shed tears, but considering that doctors ought to be cool and composed in every emergency, said coldly:

"It's a nervous breakdown. But it's nothing. Let us go at once to the doctor."

"Wherever you like, only for God's sake, make haste!"

"Don't excite yourself. You must try and control yourself."

The artist and the medical student with trembling hands put Vassilyev's coat and hat on and led him out into the street.

"Mihail Sergeyitch has been wanting to make your acquaintance for a long time," the medical student said on the way. "He is a very nice man and thoroughly good at his work. He took his degree in 1882, and he has an immense practice already. He treats students as though he were one himself."

"Make haste, make haste!" Vassilyev urged.

Mihail Sergeyitch, a stout, fair-haired doctor, received the friends with politeness and frigid dignity, and smiled only on one side of his face.

"Rybnikov and Mayer have spoken to me of your illness already," he said. "Very glad to be of service to you. Well? Sit down, I beg."

He made Vassilyev sit down in a big armchair near the table, and moved a box of cigarettes towards him.

"Now then!" he began, stroking his knees. "Let us work. How old are you?"

He asked questions and the medical student answered them. He asked whether Vassilyev's father had suffered from certain special diseases, whether he drank to excess, whether he were remarkable for cruelty or any peculiarities. He made similar inquiries about his grandfather, mother, sisters, and brothers. On learning that his mother had a beautiful voice and sometimes acted on the stage, he grew more animated at once, and asked:

"Excuse me, but don't you remember, perhaps, your mother had a passion for the stage?"

Twenty minutes passed. Vassilyev was annoyed by the way the doctor kept stroking his knees and talking of the same thing.

"So far as I understand your questions, doctor," he said, "you want to know whether my illness is hereditary or not. It is not."

The doctor proceeded to ask Vassilyev whether he had had any secret vices as a boy, or had received injuries to his head; whether he had had any aberrations, any peculiarities, or exceptional propensities. Half the questions usually asked by doctors of their patients can be left unanswered without the slightest ill effect on the health, but Mihail Sergeyitch, the medical student, and the artist all looked as though if Vassilyev failed to answer one question all would be lost. As he received answers, the doctor for some reason noted them down on a slip of paper. On learning that Vassilyev had taken his degree in natural science, and was now studying law, the doctor pondered.

"He wrote a first-rate piece of original work last year," said the medical student.

"I beg your pardon, but don't interrupt me; you prevent me from concentrating," said the doctor, and he smiled on one side of his face. "Though, of course, that does enter into the diagnosis. Intense intellectual work, nervous exhaustion. Yes, yes. And do you drink vodka?" he said, addressing Vassilyev.

Another twenty minutes passed. The medical student began telling the doctor in a low voice his opinion as to the immediate cause of the attack, and described how the day before yesterday the artist, Vassilyev, and he had visited S. Street.

The indifferent, reserved, and frigid tone in which his friends and the doctor spoke of the women and that miserable street struck Vassilyev as strange in the extreme.

"Doctor, tell me one thing only," he said, controlling himself so as not to speak rudely. "Is prostitution an evil or not?"

"My dear fellow, who disputes it?" said the doctor, with an expression that suggested that he had settled all such questions for himself long ago. "Who disputes it?"

"You are a mental doctor, aren't you?" Vassilyev asked curtly.

"Yes, a mental doctor."

"Perhaps all of you are right?" said Vassilyev, getting up and beginning to walk from one end of the room to the other. "Perhaps! But it all seems marvelous to me! That I should have taken my degree in two faculties you look upon as a great achievement; because I have written a work which in three years will be thrown aside and forgotten, I am praised up to the skies; but because I cannot speak of fallen women as unconcernedly as of these chairs, I am being examined by a doctor, I am called mad, I am pitied!"

Vassilyev for some reason felt all at once unutterably sorry for himself, and his companions, and all the people he had seen two days before, and for the doctor; he burst into tears and sank into a chair.

His friends looked inquiringly at the doctor. The latter, with the air of completely comprehending the tears and the despair, of feeling himself a specialist in that line, went up to Vassilyev and, without a word gave him some medicine to drink; and then, when he was calmer, undressed him and began to investigate the degree of sensibility of the skin, the reflex action of the knees, and so on.

And Vassilyev felt easier. When he came out from the doctor's he was beginning to feel ashamed; the rattle of the carriages no longer irritated him, and the load at his heart grew lighter as though it were melting away. He had two prescriptions in his hand: one was for bromide, one was for morphine. He had taken all these remedies before!

In the street he stood still and, saying good-by to his friends, dragged himself languidly to the University.

Ward No. 6

In the hospital yard there stands a small lodge surrounded by a perfect forest of burdocks, nettles, and wild hemp. Its roof is rusty, the chimney is tumbling down, the steps at the front door are rotting away and overgrown with grass, and there are only traces left of the stucco. The front of the lodge faces the hospital; at the back it looks out into the open country, from which it is separated by the gray hospital fence with nails on it. These nails, with their points upward, and the fence, and the lodge itself, have that peculiar, desolate, God-forsaken look which is only found in our hospital and prison buildings.

If you are not afraid of being stung by the nettles, come by the narrow footpath that leads to the lodge, and let us see what is going on inside. Opening the first door, we walk into the entry. Here along the walls and by the stove every sort of hospital rubbish lies littered about. Mattresses, old tattered dressing-gowns, trousers, blue striped shirts, boots and shoes no good for anything—all these remnants are piled up in heaps, mixed up and crumpled, moldering and giving out a sickly smell.

The porter, Nikita, an old soldier wearing rusty good-conduct stripes, is always lying on the litter with a pipe between his teeth. He has a grim, surly, battered-looking face, overhanging eyebrows that give him the expression of a sheep dog of the steppes, and a red nose; he is short and looks thin and scraggy, but he is of imposing deportment and his fists are vigorous. He belongs to the class of simple-hearted, practical, and dull-witted people, prompt in carrying out orders, who like discipline better than anything in the world, and so are convinced that it is their duty to beat people. He showers blows on the face, on the chest, on the back, on whatever comes first, and is convinced that there would be no order in the place if he did not.

Next you come into a big, spacious room, which fills up the whole lodge except for the entry. Here the walls are painted a dirty blue, the ceiling is as sooty as in a hut without a chimney—it is evident that in the winter the stove smokes and the room is full of fumes. The windows are disfigured by iron gratings on the inside. The wooden floor is gray and full of splinters. There is a stench of sour cabbage, of smoldering wicks, of bugs, and of ammonia, and for the first minute this stench gives you the impression of having walked into a menagerie.

There are bedsteads screwed to the floor. Men in blue hospital dressing gowns, and wearing night-caps in the old style, are sitting and lying on them. These are the lunatics.

There are five of them in all here. Only one is of the upper class, the rest are all artisans. The one nearest the door—a tall, lean workman with shining red whiskers and tear-stained eyes—sits with his head propped on his hand, staring at the same point. Day and night he grieves, shaking his head, sighing and smiling bitterly. He rarely takes a part in conversation and usually makes no answer to questions; he eats and drinks mechanically when food is offered him. From his agonizing, throbbing cough, his thinness, and the flush of his cheeks, one may judge that he is in the first stage of consumption. Next to him is a little, alert, very lively old man, with a pointed beard and curly black hair like a Negro's. By day he walks up and down the ward from window to window, or sits on his bed, cross-legged like a Turk, and, ceaselessly as a bullfinch whistles, softly sings and titters. He shows his childish gaiety and lively character at night also when he gets up to say his prayers—that is, to beat himself on the chest with his fists, and to scratch with his fingers at the door. This is the Jew Moiseika, an imbecile, who went crazy twenty years ago when his hat factory was burnt down.

And of all the inhabitants of Ward No. 6, he is the only one who is allowed to go out of the lodge, and even out of the yard into the street. He has enjoyed this privilege for years, probably because he is an old inhabitant of the hospital—a quiet, harmless imbecile, the buffoon of the town, where people are used to seeing him surrounded by boys and dogs. In his wretched gown, in his absurd nightcap and in slippers, sometimes with bare legs and even without trousers, he walks about the streets, stopping at the gates and little shops, and begging for a copper. In one place they will give him some kvass, in another some bread, in another a copper, so that he generally goes back to the ward feeling rich and well fed. Everything that he brings back Nikita takes from him for his own benefit. The soldier does this roughly, angrily turning the Jew's pockets inside out, and calling God to witness that he will not let him go into the street again, and that breach of the regulations is worse to him than anything in the world.

Moiseika likes to make himself useful. He gives his companions water, and covers them up when they are asleep; he promises each of them to bring him back a kopeck, and to make him a new cap; he feeds with a spoon his neighbor on the left, who is paralyzed. He acts in this way, not from compassion or from any considerations of a humane kind, but through imitation, unconsciously dominated by Gromov, his neighbor on the right hand.

Ivan Dmitritch Gromov, a man of thirty-three, who is a gentleman by birth, and has been a court usher and provincial secretary, suffers from the mania of persecution. He either lies curled up in bed, or walks from corner to corner as though for exercise; he very rarely sits down. He is always excited, agitated, and overwrought by a sort of vague, undefined expectation. The faintest rustle in the entry or shout in the yard is enough to make him raise his head and begin listening: whether they are coming for him, whether they are looking for him. And at such times his face expresses the utmost uneasiness and repulsion.

I like his broad face with its high cheekbones, always pale and unhappy, and reflecting, as though in a mirror, a soul tormented by conflict and long-continued terror. His grimaces are strange and abnormal, but the delicate lines traced on his face by profound, genuine suffering show intelligence and sense, and there is a warm and healthy light in his eyes. I like the man himself, courteous, anxious to be of use, and extraordinarily gentle to everyone except Nikita. When anyone drops a button or a spoon, he jumps up from his bed quickly and picks it up; every day he says good-morning to his companions, and when he goes to bed he wishes them goodnight.

Besides his continually overwrought condition and his grimaces, his madness shows itself in the following way also. Sometimes in the evenings he wraps himself in his dressing-gown, and, trembling all over, with his teeth chattering, begins walking rapidly from corner to corner and between the bedsteads. It seems as though he is in a violent fever. From the way he suddenly stops and glances at his companions, it can be seen that he is longing to say something very important, but, apparently reflecting that they would not listen, or would not understand him, he shakes his head impatiently and goes on pacing up and down. But soon the desire to speak gets the upper hand of every consideration, and he will let himself go and speak fervently and passionately. His talk is disordered and feverish like delirium, disconnected, and not always intelligible, but, on the other hand, something extremely fine may be felt in it, both in the words and the voice. When he talks you recognize in him the lunatic and the man. It is difficult to reproduce on paper his insane talk. He speaks of the baseness of mankind, of violence trampling on justice, of the glorious life, which will one day be upon earth, of the window-gratings, which remind him every minute of the stupidity and cruelty of oppressors. It makes a disorderly, incoherent potpourri of themes old but not yet out of date.

II

Some twelve or fifteen years ago an official called Gromov, a highly respectable and prosperous person, was living in his own house in the principal street of the town. He had two sons, Sergey and Ivan. When Sergey was a student in his fourth year he was taken ill with galloping consumption and died, and his death was, as it were, the first of a whole series of calamities that suddenly showered on the

Gromov family. Within a week of Sergey's funeral the old father was put on his trial for fraud and misappropriation, and he died of typhoid in the prison hospital soon afterwards. The house, with all their belongings, was sold by auction, and Ivan Dmitritch and his mother were left entirely without means.

Hitherto in his father's lifetime, Ivan Dmitritch, who was studying in the University of Petersburg, had received an allowance of sixty or seventy rubles a month, and had had no conception of poverty; now he had to make an abrupt change in his life. He had to spend his time from morning to night giving lessons for next to nothing, to work at copying, and with all that to go hungry, as all his earnings were sent to keep his mother. Ivan Dmitritch could not stand such a life; he lost heart and strength, and, giving up the university, went home.

Here, through interest, he obtained the post of teacher in the district school, but could not get on with his colleagues, was not liked by the boys, and soon gave up the post. His mother died. He was for six months without work, living on nothing but bread and water; then he became a court usher. He kept his post until he was dismissed owing to his illness.

He had never even in his young student days given the impression of being perfectly healthy. He had always been pale, thin, and given to catching cold; he ate little and slept badly. A single glass of wine went to his head and made him hysterical. He always had a craving for society, but, owing to his irritable temperament and suspiciousness, he never became very intimate with anyone, and had no friends. He always spoke with contempt of his fellow-townsmen, saying that their coarse ignorance and sleepy animal existence seemed to him loathsome and horrible. He spoke in a loud tenor, with heat, and invariably either with scorn and indignation, or with wonder and enthusiasm, and always with perfect sincerity. Whatever one talked to him about, he always brought it round to the same subject: that life was dull and stifling in the town; that the townspeople had no lofty interests, but lived a dingy, meaningless life, diversified by violence, coarse profligacy, and hypocrisy; that scoundrels were well fed and clothed, while honest men lived from hand to mouth; that they needed schools, a progressive local paper, a theatre, public lectures, the co-ordination of the intellectual elements; that society must see its failings and be horrified. In his criticisms of people he laid on the colors thick using only black and white, and no fine shades; mankind was divided for him into honest men and scoundrels: there was nothing in between. He always spoke with passion and enthusiasm of women and of love, but he had never been in love.

In spite of the severity of his judgments and his nervousness, he was liked, and behind his back was spoken of affectionately as Vanya. His innate refinement and readiness to be of service, his good breeding, his moral purity, and his shabby coat, his frail appearance and family misfortunes, aroused a kind, warm, sorrow-ful feeling. Moreover, he was well educated and well read; according to the towns-people's notions, he knew everything, and was in their eyes something like a walk-ing encyclopedia.

He had read a great deal. He would sit at the club, nervously pulling at his beard and looking through the magazines and books; and from his face one could see that he was not reading, but devouring the pages without giving himself time to digest what he read. It must be supposed that reading was one of his morbid habits, as he fell upon anything that came into his hands with equal avidity, even last year's newspapers and calendars. At home he always read lying down.

III

One autumn morning Ivan Dmitritch, turning up the collar of his greatcoat and splashing through the mud, made his way by side streets and back lanes to see some artisan, and to collect some payment that was owed. He was in a gloomy mood, as he always was in the morning. In one of the side streets he was met by two convicts in fetters and four soldiers with rifles in charge of them. Ivan Dmitritch had very often met convicts before, and they had always excited feel-ings of compassion and discomfort in him; but now this meeting made a pecu-liar, strange impression on him. It suddenly seemed to him for some reason that he, too, might be put into fetters and led through the mud to prison like that. After visiting the artisan, on the way home he met near the post office a police superintendent of his acquaintance, who greeted him and walked a few paces along the street with him, and for some reason this seemed to him suspicious. At home he could not get the convicts or the soldiers with their rifles out of his head all day, and an unaccountable inward agitation prevented him from read-ing or concentrating his mind. In the evening he did not light his lamp, and at night he could not sleep, but kept thinking that he might be arrested, put into fetters, and thrown into prison. He did not know of any harm he had done, and could be certain that he would never be guilty of murder, arson, or theft in the future either; but was it not easy to commit a crime by accident, unconsciously, and was not false witness always possible, and indeed, miscarriage of justice? It was not without good reason that the age long experience of the simple people teaches that beggary and prison are ills none can be safe from. A judicial mis-take is very possible as legal proceedings are conducted nowadays, and there is nothing to be wondered at in it. People who have an official, professional rela-tion to other men's sufferings—for instance, judges, police officers, doctors—in course of time, through habit, grow so callous that they cannot, even if they wish it, take any but a formal attitude to their clients; in this respect they are not different from the peasant who slaughters sheep and calves in the back-yard, and does not notice the blood. With this formal, soulless attitude to human personality the judge needs but one thing—time—in order to deprive an innocent man of all rights of property, and to condemn him to penal servitude. Only the time spent on performing certain formalities for which the judge is paid his salary, and then—it is all over. Then you may look in vain for justice and protection in this dirty, wretched little town a hundred and fifty miles from a railway station! And, indeed, is it not absurd even to think of justice when every kind of violence is accepted by society as a rational and consistent necessity, and every act of mercy—for instance, a verdict of acquittal—calls forth a perfect outburst of dissatisfied and revengeful feeling?

In the morning Ivan Dmitritch got up from his bed in a state of horror, with cold perspiration on his forehead, completely convinced that he might be arrested any minute. Since his gloomy thoughts of yesterday had haunted him so long, he thought, it must be that there was some truth in them. They could not, indeed, have come into his mind without any grounds whatever.

A policeman walking slowly passed by the windows: that was not for nothing. Here were two men standing still and silent near the house. Why were they silent? And agonizing days and nights followed for Ivan Dmitritch. Everyone who passed by the windows or came into the yard seemed to him a spy or a detective. At midday the chief of the police usually drove down the street with a pair of horses; he was going from his estate near the town to the police department; but Ivan Dmitritch fancied every time that he was driving especially quickly, and that he had a peculiar expression: it was evident that he was in haste to announce that there was a very important criminal in the town. Ivan Dmitritch started at every ring at the bell and knock at the gate, and was agitated whenever he came upon anyone new at his landlady's; when he met police officers and gendarmes he smiled and began whistling so as to seem unconcerned. He could not sleep for whole nights in succession expecting to be arrested, but he snored loudly and sighed as though in deep sleep that his landlady might think he was asleep; for if he could not sleep it meant that he was tormented by the stings of conscience—what a piece of evidence! Facts and common sense persuaded him that all these terrors were nonsense and morbidity, that if one looked at the matter more broadly there was nothing really terrible in arrest and imprisonment—so long as the conscience is at ease; but more sensibly and logically he reasoned, the more acute and agonizing his mental distress became. It might be compared with the story of a hermit who tried to cut a dwelling-place for himself in a virgin forest; the more zealously he worked with his axe the thicker the forest grew. In the end Ivan Dmitritch, seeing it was useless, gave up reasoning altogether, and abandoned himself entirely to despair and terror.

He began to avoid people and to seek solitude. His official work had been distasteful to him before: now it became unbearable to him. He was afraid they would somehow get him into trouble, would put a bribe in his pocket unnoticed and then denounce him, or that he would accidentally make a mistake in official papers that would appear to be fraudulent, or would lose other people's money. It is strange that his imagination had never at other times been so agile and inventive as now, when every day he thought of thousands of different reasons for being seriously anxious over his freedom and honor; but, on the other hand, his interest in the outer world, in books in particular, grew sensibly fainter, and his memory began to fail him.

In the spring when the snow melted there were found in the ravine near the cemetery two half-decomposed corpses—the bodies of an old woman and a boy bearing the traces of death by violence. Nothing was talked of but these bodies and their unknown murderers. That people might not think he had been guilty of the crime, Ivan Dmitritch walked about the streets, smiling, and when he met acquaintances he turned pale, flushed, and began declaring that there was no greater crime than the murder of the weak and defenseless. But this duplicity soon exhausted him, and after some reflection he decided that in his position the best thing to do was to hide in his landlady's cellar. He sat in the cellar all day and then all night, then another day, was fearfully cold, and waiting till dusk, stole secretly like a thief back to his room. He stood in the middle of the room till daybreak, listening without stirring. Very early in the morning, before sunrise, some workmen came into the house. Ivan Dmitritch knew perfectly well that they had come to mend the stove in the kitchen, but terror told him that they were police officers disguised as workmen. He slipped stealthily out of the flat, and, overcome by terror, ran along the street without his cap and coat. Dogs raced after him barking, a peasant shouted somewhere behind him, the wind whistled in his ears, and it seemed to Ivan Dmitritch that the force and violence of the whole world was massed together behind his back and was chasing after him.

He was stopped and brought home, and his landlady sent for a doctor. Doctor Andrey Yefimitch, of whom we shall have more to say hereafter, prescribed cold compresses on his head and laurel drops, shook his head, and went away, telling the landlady he should not come again, as one should not interfere with people who are going out of their minds. As he had not the means to live at home and be nursed, Ivan Dmitritch was soon sent to the hospital, and was there put into the ward for venereal patients. He could not sleep at night, was full of whims and fancies, and disturbed by patients, and was soon afterwards, by Andrey Yefimitch's orders, transferred to Ward No. 6.

Within a year Ivan Dmitritch was completely forgotten in the town, and his books, heaped up by his landlady in a sledge in the shed, were pulled to pieces by boys.

IV

Ivan Dmitritch's neighbor on the left hand is, as I have said already, the Jew Moiseika; his neighbor on the right hand is a peasant so rolling in fat that he is almost spherical, with a blankly stupid face, utterly devoid of thought. This is a motionless, gluttonous, unclean animal who has long ago lost all powers of thought or feeling. An acrid, stifling stench always comes from him.

Nikita, who has to clean up after him, beats him terribly with all his might not sparing his fists; and what is dreadful is not his being beaten—but the fact that this stupefied creature does not respond to the blows with a sound or a movement, nor by a look in the eyes, but only sways a little like a heavy barrel.

The fifth and last inhabitant of Ward No. 6 is a man of the artisan class who has once been a sorter in the post office, a thinnish, fair little man with a good-natured but rather sly face. To judge from the clear, cheerful look in his calm and intelligent eyes, he has some pleasant idea in his mind, and has some very important and agreeable secret. He has under his pillow and under his mattress something that he never shows anyone, not from fear of its being taken from him and stolen, but from modesty. Sometimes he goes to the window, and turning his back to his companions, puts something on his breast, and bending his head, looks at it; if you go up to him at such a moment, he is overcome with confusion and snatches something off his breast. But it is not difficult to guess his secret.

"Congratulate me," he often says to Ivan Dmitritch; "I have been presented with the Stanislav order of the second degree with the star. The second degree with the star is only given to foreigners, but for some reason they want to make an exception for me," he says with a smile, shrugging his shoulders in perplexity. "That I must confess I did not expect."

"I don't understand anything about that," Ivan Dmitritch replies morosely.

"But do you know what I shall attain to sooner or later?" the former sorter persists, screwing up his eyes slyly. "I shall certainly get the Swedish 'Polar Star.' That's an order it is worth working for, a white cross with a black ribbon. It's very beautiful."

Probably in no other place is life so monotonous as in this ward. In the morning the patients, except the paralytic and the fat peasant, wash in the entry at a big tub and wipe themselves with the skirts of their dressing gowns; after that they drink tea out of tin mugs that Nikita brings them out of the main building. Everyone is allowed one mugful. At midday they have soup made out of sour cabbage and boiled grain, in the evening their supper consists of grain left from dinner. In the intervals they lie down, sleep, look out of window, and walk from one corner to the other. And so every day. Even the former sorter always talks of the same orders.

Fresh faces are rarely seen in Ward No. 6. The doctor has not taken in any new mental cases for a long time, and the people who are fond of visiting lunatic asylums are few in this world. Once every two months Semyon Lazaritch, the barber, appears in the ward. How he cuts the patients' hair, and how Nikita helps him to do it, and what a trepidation the lunatics are always thrown into by the arrival of the drunken, smiling barber, we will not describe.

No one even looks into the ward except the barber. The patients are condemned to see day after day no one but Nikita.

A rather strange rumor has, however, been circulating in the hospital of late. It is rumored that the doctor has begun to visit Ward No. 6.

V

A strange rumor!

Dr. Andrey Yefimitch Ragin is a strange man in his way. They say that when he was young he was very religious, and prepared himself for a clerical career, and that when he had finished his studies at the high school in 1863 he intended to enter a theological academy, but that his father, a surgeon and doctor of medicine, jeered at him and declared point-blank that he would disown him if he became a priest. How far this is true I don't know, but Andrey Yefimitch himself has more than once confessed that he has never had a natural bent for medicine or science in general.

However that may have been, when he finished his studies in the medical faculty he did not enter the priesthood. He showed no special devoutness, and was no more like a priest at the beginning of his medical career than he is now.

His exterior is heavy, coarse like a peasant's, his face, his beard, his flat hair, and his coarse, clumsy figure, suggest an overfed, intemperate, and harsh innkeeper on the highroad. His face is surly-looking and covered with blue veins, his eyes are little and his nose is red. With his height and broad shoulders he has huge hands and feet; one would think that a blow from his fist would knock the life out of anyone, but his step is soft, and his walk is cautious and insinuating; when he meets anyone in a narrow passage he is always the first to stop and make way, and to say, not in a bass, as one would expect, but in a high, soft tenor: "I beg your pardon!" He has little swelling on his neck, which prevents him from wearing stiff starched collars, and so he always goes about in soft linen or cotton shirts. Altogether he does not dress like a doctor. He wears the same suit for ten years, and the new clothes, which he usually buys at a Jewish shop, look shabby and crumpled on him as his old ones; he sees patients and dines and pays visits all in the same coat; but this is not due to niggardliness, but to complete carelessness about his appearance.

When Andrey Yefimitch came to the town to take up his duties the "institution founded for the glory of God" was in a terrible condition. One could hardly breathe for the stench in the wards, in the passages, and in the courtyards of the hospital. The hospital servants, the nurses, and their children slept in the wards together with the patients. They complained that there was no living for beetles, bugs, and mice. The surgical wards were never free from erysipelas. There were only two scalpels and not one thermometer in the whole hospital; potatoes were kept in baths. The superintendent, the housekeeper, and the medical assistant robbed the patients, and of the old doctor, Andrey Yefimitch's predecessor, people declared that he secretly sold the hospital alcohol, and that he kept a regular harem consisting of nurses and female patients. These disorderly proceedings were perfectly well known in the town, and were even exaggerated, but people took them calmly; some justified them on the ground that there were only peasants and working men in the hospital, who could not be dissatisfied, since they were much worse off at home than in the hospital—they couldn't be fed on woodcocks! Others said in excuse that the town alone, without help from the Zemstvo, was not equal to maintaining a good hospital; thank God for having one at all, even a poor one. And the newly formed Zemstvo did not open infirmaries either in the town or the neighborhood, relying on the fact that the town already had its hospital.

After looking over the hospital Andrey Yefimitch came to the conclusion that it was an immoral institution and extremely prejudicial to the health of the townspeople. In his opinion the most sensible thing that could be done was to let out the patients and close the hospital. But he reflected that his will alone was not enough to do this, and that it would be useless; if physical and moral impurity were driven out of one place, they would only move to another; one must wait for it to wither away of itself. Besides, if people open a hospital and put up with having it, it must be because they need it; superstition and all the nastiness and abominations of daily life were necessary, since in process of time they worked out to something sensible, just as manure turns into black earth. There was nothing on earth so good that it had not something nasty about its first origin.

When Andrey Yefimitch undertook his duties he was apparently not greatly concerned about the irregularities at the hospital. He only asked the attendants and nurses not to sleep in the wards, and had two cupboards of instruments put up; the superintendent, the housekeeper, the medical assistant, and the erysipelas remained unchanged.

Andrey Yefimitch loved intelligence and honesty intensely, but he had no strength of will nor belief in his right to organize an intelligent and honest life about him. He was absolutely unable to give orders, to forbid things, and to insist. It seemed as though he had taken a vow never to raise his voice and never to make use of the imperative. It was difficult for him to say "Fetch" or "Bring"; when he wanted his meals he would cough hesitatingly and say to the cook: "How about tea?" or "How about dinner?" To dismiss the superintendent or to tell him to leave off stealing, or to abolish the unnecessary parasitic post altogether, was absolutely beyond his powers. When Andrey Yefimitch was deceived or flattered, or accounts he knew to be cooked were brought him to sign, he would turn as red as a crab and feel guilty, but yet he would sign the accounts. When the patients complained to him of being hungry or of the roughness of the nurses, he would be confused and mutter guiltily: "Very well, very well, I will go into it later. . . . Most likely there is some misunderstanding. . . ."

At first Andrey Yefimitch worked very zealously. He saw patients every day from morning till dinnertime, performed operations, and even attended confinements. The ladies said of him that he was attentive and clever at diagnosing diseases, especially those of women and children. But in process of time the work unmistakably wearied him by its monotony and obvious uselessness. Today one sees thirty patients, and tomorrow they have increased to thirty-five, the next day forty, and so on from day to day, from year to year, while the mortality in the town did not decrease and the patients did not leave off coming. To be any real help to forty patients between morning and dinner was not physically possible, so it could but lead to deception. If twelve thousand patients were seen in a year it meant, if one looked at it simply that twelve thousand men were deceived. To put those who were seriously ill into wards, and to treat them according to the principles of science, was impossible, too, because though there were principles there was no science; if he were to put aside philosophy and pedantically follow the rules as other doctors did, the things above all necessary were cleanliness and ventilation instead of dirt, wholesome nourishment instead of broth made of stinking, sour cabbage, and good assistants instead of thieves; and, indeed, why hinder people dying if death is the normal and legitimate end of everyone? What is gained if some shopkeeper or clerk lives an extra five or ten years? If the aim of medicine is by drugs to alleviate suffering, the question forces itself on one: why alleviate it? In the first place, they say that suffering leads man to perfection; and in the second, if mankind really learns to alleviate its sufferings with pills and drops, it will completely abandon religion and philosophy, in which it has hitherto found not merely protection from all sorts of trouble, but even happiness. Pushkin suffered terrible agonies before his death, poor Heine lay paralyzed for several years; why, then should not some Andrey Yefimitch or Matryona Savishna be ill, since their lives had nothing of importance in them, and would have been entirely empty and like the life of an amoeba except for suffering?

Oppressed by such reflections, Andrey Yefimitch relaxed his efforts and gave up visiting the hospital every day.

VI

His life was passed like this. As a rule he got up at eight o'clock in the morning, dressed, and drank his tea. Then he sat down in his study to read, or went to the hospital. At the hospital the out-patients were sitting in the dark, narrow little corridor waiting to be seen by the doctor. The nurses and the attendants, tramping with their boots over the brick floors, ran by them; gaunt-looking patients in dressing-gowns passed; dead bodies and vessels full of filth were carried by; the children were crying, and there was a cold draught. Andrey Yefimitch knew that such surroundings were torture to feverish, consumptive, and impressionable patients; but what could be done? In the consulting-room he was met by his assistant, Sergey Sergeyitch—a fat little man with a plump, well-washed shaven face, with soft, smooth manners, wearing a new loosely cut suit, and looking more like a senator than a medical assistant. He had an immense practice in the town, wore a white tie, and considered himself more proficient than the doctor, who had no practice. In the corner of the consulting-room there stood a huge icon in a shrine with a heavy lamp in front of it, and near it a candle-stand with a white cover on it. On the walls hung portraits of bishops, a view of the Svyatogorsky Monastery, and wreaths of dried cornflowers. Sergey Sergeyitch was religious, and liked solemnity and decorum. The icon had been put up at his expense; at his instructions some one of the patients read the hymns of praise in the consulting-room on Sundays, and after the reading Sergey Sergeyitch himself went through the wards with a censer and burned incense.

There were a great many patients, but the time was short, and so the work was confined to the asking of a few brief questions and the administration of some drugs, such as castor-oil or volatile ointment. Andrey Yefimitch would sit with his cheek resting in his hand, lost in thought and asking questions mechanically. Sergey Sergeyitch sat down too, rubbing his hands, and from time to time putting in his word.

"We suffer pain and poverty," he would say, "because we do not pray to the merciful God as we should. Yes!"

Andrey Yefimitch never performed any operations when he was seeing patients; he had long ago given up doing so, and the sight of blood upset him. When he had to open a child's mouth in order to look at its throat, and the child cried and tried to defend itself with its little hands, the noise in his ears made his head go round and brought tears into his eyes. He would make haste to prescribe a drug, and motion to the woman to take the child away.

He was soon wearied by the timidity of the patients and their incoherence, by the proximity of the pious Sergey Sergeyitch, by the portraits on the walls, and by his own questions, which he had asked over and over again for twenty years. And he would go away after seeing five or six patients. The rest would be seen by his assistant in his absence.

With the agreeable thought that, thank God, he had no private practice now, and that no one would interrupt him, Andrey Yefimitch sat down to the table immediately on reaching home and took up a book. He read a great deal and always with enjoyment. Half his salary went on buying books, and of the six rooms that made up his abode three were heaped up with books and old magazines. He liked best of all works on history and philosophy; the only medical publication to which he subscribed was *The Doctor,* of which he always read the last pages first. He would always go on reading for several hours without a break and without being weary. He did not read as rapidly and impulsively as Ivan Dmitritch had done in the past, but slowly and with concentration, often pausing over a passage, which he liked or did not find intelligible. Near the books there always stood a decanter of vodka, and a salted cucumber or a pickled apple lay beside it, not on a plate, but on the baize tablecloth. Every half-hour he would pour himself out a glass of vodka and drink it without taking his eyes off the book. Then without looking at it he would feel for the cucumber and bite off a bit.

At three o'clock he would go cautiously to the kitchen door, cough, and say: "Daryushka, what about dinner?"

After his dinner—a rather poor and untidily served one—Andrey Yefimitch would walk up and down his rooms with his arms folded, thinking. The clock would strike four, then five, and still he would be walking up and down thinking. Occasionally the kitchen door would creak, and the red and sleepy face of Daryushka would appear.

"Andrey Yefimitch, isn't it time for you to have your beer?" she would ask anxiously.

"No, it is not time yet. . . ." he would answer. "I'll wait a little . . . I'll wait a little."

Towards the evening the postmaster, Mihail Averyanitch, the only man in the town whose society did not bore Andrey Yefimitch, would come in. Mihail Averyanitch had once been a very rich landowner and had served in the cavalry, but had come to ruin, and was forced by poverty to take a job in the post office late in life. He had a hale and hearty appearance, luxuriant gray whiskers, the manners of a well-bred man, and a loud, pleasant voice. He was good-natured and emotional, but hot-tempered. When anyone in the post office made a protest, expressed disagreement, or even began to argue, Mihail Averyanitch would turn crimson, shake all over, and shout in a voice of thunder, "Hold your tongue!" so that the post office had long enjoyed the reputation of an institution which it was terrible to visit. Mihail Averyanitch liked and respected Andrey Yefimitch for his culture and the loftiness of his soul; he treated the other inhabitants of the town superciliously, as though they were his subordinates.

"Here I am," he would say, going into Andrey Yefimitch. "Good-evening, my dear fellow! I'll be bound, you are getting sick of me, aren't you!"

"On the contrary, I am delighted," said the doctor. "I am always glad to see you."

The friends would sit down on the sofa in the study and for some time would smoke in silence.

"Daryushka, what about the beer?" Andrey Yefimitch would say.

They would drink their first bottle still in silence, the doctor brooding and Mihail Averyanitch with a gay and animated face, like a man who has something very interesting to tell. The doctor was always the one to begin the conversation.

"What a pity," he would say quietly and slowly, not looking his friend in the face (he never looked anyone in the face)—"what a great pity it is that there are no people in our town who are capable of carrying on intelligent and interesting conversation, or care to do so. It is an immense privation for us. Even the educated class do not rise above vulgarity; the level of their development, I assure you, is not a bit higher than that of the lower orders."

"Perfectly true. I agree"

"You know, of course," the doctor went on quietly and deliberately, "that everything in this world is insignificant and uninteresting except the higher spiritual manifestations of the human mind. Intellect draws a sharp line between the animals and man, suggests the divinity of the latter, and to some extent even takes the place of the immortality which does not exist. Consequently, the intellect is the only possible source of enjoyment. We see and hear of no trace of intellect about us, so we are deprived of enjoyment. We have books, it is true, but that is not at all the same as living talk and converse. If you will allow me to make a not quite apt comparison: books are the printed score, while talk is the singing."

"Perfectly true."

A silence would follow. Daryushka would come out of the kitchen and with an expression of blank dejection would stand in the doorway to listen, with her face propped on her fist.

"Eh!" Mihail Averyanitch would sigh. "To expect intelligence of this generation!"

And he would describe how wholesome, entertaining, and interesting life had been in the past. How intelligent the educated class in Russia used to be, and what lofty ideas it had of honor and friendship; how they used to lend money without an IOU, and it was thought a disgrace not to give a helping hand to a comrade in need; and what campaigns, what adventures, what skirmishes, what comrades, what women! And the Caucasus, what a marvelous country! The wife of a battalion commander, a queer woman, used to put on an officer's uniform and drive off into the mountains in the evening, alone, without a guide. It was said that she had a love affair with some princeling in the native village.

"Queen of Heaven, Holy Mother," Daryushka would sigh.

"And how we drank! And how we ate! And what desperate liberals we were!"

Andrey Yefimitch would listen without hearing; he was musing as he sipped his beer.

"I often dream of intellectual people and conversation with them," he said suddenly, interrupting Mihail Averyanitch. "My father gave me an excellent education, but under the influence of the ideas of the sixties made me become a doctor. I believe if I had not obeyed him then, by now I should have been in the very center of the intellectual movement. Most likely I should have become a member of some university. Of course, intellect, too, is transient and not eternal, but you know why I cherish a partiality for it. Life is a vexatious trap; when a thinking man reaches maturity and attains to full consciousness he cannot help feeling that he is in a trap from which there is no escape. Indeed, he is summoned without his choice of fortuitous circumstances from non-existence into life ... what for? He tries to find out the meaning and object of his existence; he is told nothing, or he is told absurdities; he knocks and it is not opened to him; death comes to him—also without his choice. And so, just as in prison men held together by common misfortune feel more at ease when they are together, so one does not notice the trap in life when people with a bent for analysis and generalization meet together and pass their time in the interchange of proud and free ideas. In that sense the intellect is the source of an enjoyment nothing can replace."

"Perfectly true."

Not looking his friend in the face Andrey Yefimitch would go on, quietly and with pauses, talking about intellectual people and conversation with them, and Mihail Averyanitch would listen attentively and agree: "Perfectly true."

"And you do not believe in the immortality of the soul?" he would ask suddenly.

"No, honored Mihail Averyanitch; I do not believe it, and have no grounds for believing it."

"I must own I doubt it too. And yet I have a feeling as though I should never die. Oh, I think to myself: 'Old fogey, it is time you were dead!' But there is a little voice in my soul that says: 'Don't believe it; you won't die.'"

Soon after nine o'clock Mihail Averyanitch would go away. As he put on his fur coat in the entry he would say with a sigh:

"What a wilderness fate has carried us to, though, really! What's most vexatious of all is to have to die here. Ech!"

VII

After seeing his friend out Andrey Yefimitch would sit down at the table and begin reading again. The stillness of the evening, and afterwards of the night, was not broken by a single sound, and it seemed as though time were standing still and brooding with the doctor over the book, and as though there were nothing in existence but the books and the lamp with the green shade. The doctor's coarse peasant-like face was gradually lighted up by a smile of delight and enthusiasm over the progress of the human intellect. Oh, why is not man immortal? He thought. What is the good of the brain centers and convolutions, what is the good of sight, speech, self-consciousness, genius, if it is all destined to depart into the soil, and in the end to grow cold together with the earth's crust, and then for millions of years, to fly with the earth round the sun with no meaning and no object? To do that there was no need at all to draw man with his lofty, almost godlike intellect out of non-existence, and then, as though in mockery, to turn him into clay. The transmutation of substances! But what cowardice to comfort oneself with that cheap substitute for immortality! The unconscious processes that take place in nature are lower even than the stupidity of man, since in stupidity there is, anyway, consciousness and will, while in those processes there is absolutely nothing. Only the coward who has more fear of death than dignity can comfort himself with the fact that his body will in time live again in the grass, in the stones, in the toad. To find one's immortality in the transmutation of substances is as strange as to prophesy a brilliant future for the case after a precious violin has been broken and become useless.

When the clock struck, Andrey Yefimitch would sink back into his chair and close his eyes to think a little. And under the influence of the fine ideas of which he had been reading he would, unawares, recall his past and his present. The past was hateful—better not to think of it. And it was the same in the present as in the past. He knew that at the very time when his thoughts were floating together with the cooling earth round the sun, in the main building beside his abode people were suffering in sickness and physical impurity: someone perhaps could not sleep and was making war upon the insects, someone was being infected by erysipelas, or moaning over too tight a bandage; perhaps the patients were playing cards with the nurses and drinking vodka. According to the yearly return, twelve thousand people had been deceived; the whole hospital rested as it had done twenty years ago on thieving, filth, scandals, gossip, on gross quackery, and, as before, it was an immoral institution extremely injurious to the health of the inhabitants. He knew that Nikita knocked the patients about behind the barred windows of Ward No. 6, and that Moiseika went about the town every day begging alms.

On the other hand, he knew very well that a magical change had taken place in medicine during the last twenty-five years. When he was studying at the university he had fancied that medicine would soon be overtaken by the fate of alchemy and metaphysics; but now when he was reading at night the science of medicine touched him and excited his wonder and even enthusiasm. What unexpected brilliance, what a revolution! Thanks to the antiseptic system operations were performed such as the great Pirogov had considered impossible even *in spe.* Ordinary Zemstvo doctors were venturing to perform the resection of the kneecap; of abdominal operations only one percent was fatal; while stone was considered such a trifle that they did not even write about it. A radical cure for syphilis had been discovered. And the theory of heredity, hypnotism, the discoveries of Pasteur and of Koch, hygiene based on statistics, and the work of our Zemstvo doctors!

Psychiatry with its modern classification of mental diseases, methods of diagnosis, and treatment, was a perfect Elborus in comparison with what had been in the past. They no longer poured cold water on the heads of lunatics nor put straitwaistcoats upon them; they treated them with humanity, and even, so it was stated in the papers, got up balls and entertainments for them. Andrey Yefimitch knew that with modern tastes and views such an abomination as Ward No. 6 was possible only a hundred and fifty miles from a railway in a little town where the mayor and all the town council were half-illiterate tradesmen who looked upon the doctor as an oracle who must be believed without any criticism even if he had poured molten lead into their mouths; in any other place the public and the newspapers would long ago have torn this little Bastille to pieces.

"But, after all, what of it?" Andrey Yefimitch would ask himself, opening his eyes. "There is the antiseptic system, there is Koch, there is Pasteur, but the essential reality is not altered a bit; ill-health and mortality are still the same. They get up balls and entertainments for the mad, but still they don't let them go free; so it's all nonsense and vanity, and there is no difference in reality between the best Vienna clinic and my hospital." But depression and a feeling akin to envy prevented him from feeling indifferent; it must have been owing to exhaustion. His heavy head sank on to the book, he put his hands under his face to make it softer, and thought: "I serve in a pernicious institution and receive a salary from people whom I am deceiving. I am not honest, but then, I of myself am nothing, I am only part of an inevitable social evil: all local officials are pernicious and receive their salary for doing nothing. . . . And so for my dishonesty it is not I who am to blame, but the times. If I had been born two hundred years later I should have been different."

When it struck three he would put out his lamp and go into his bedroom; he was not sleepy.

VIII

Two years before, the Zemstvo in a liberal mood had decided to allow three hundred rubles a year to pay for additional medical service in the town till the Zemstvo hospital should be opened, and the district doctor, Yevgeny Fyodoritch Hobotov, was invited to the town to assist Andrey Yefimitch. He was a very young man—not yet thirty—tall and dark, with broad cheek-bones and little eyes; his forefathers had probably come from one of the many alien races of Russia. He arrived in the town without a farthing, with a small portmanteau, and a plain young woman whom he called his cook. This woman had a baby at the breast. Yevgeny Fyodoritch used to go about in a cap with a peak, and in high boots, and in the winter wore a sheepskin. He made great friends with Sergey Sergeyitch, the medical assistant, and with the treasurer, but held aloof from the other officials, and for some reason called them aristocrats. He had only one book in his lodgings, "The Latest Prescriptions of the Vienna Clinic for 1881." When he went to a patient he always took this book with him. He played billiards in the evening at the club: he did not like cards. He was very fond of using in conversation such expressions as "endless bobbery," "canting soft soap," "shut up with your finicking."

He visited the hospital twice a week, made the round of the wards, and saw out-patients. The complete absence of the antiseptic treatment and the cupping roused his indignation, but he did not introduce any new system, being afraid of offending Andrey Yefimitch. He regarded his colleague as a sly old rascal, suspected him of being a man of large means, and secretly envied him. He would have been very glad to have his post.

IX

On a spring evening towards the end of March, when there was no snow left on the ground and the starlings were singing in the hospital garden, the doctor went out to see his friend the postmaster as far as the gate. At that very moment the Jew Moiseika, returning with his boot, came into the yard. He had no cap on, and his bare feet were thrust into galoshes; in his hand he had a little bag of coppers.

"Give me a kopeck!" he said to the doctor, smiling, and shivering with cold. Andrey Yefimitch, who could never refuse anyone anything, gave him a ten-kopeck piece.

"How bad that is!" he thought, looking at the Jew's bare feet with their thin red ankles.

"Why, it's wet."

And stirred by a feeling akin both to pity and disgust he went into the lodge behind the Jew, looking now at his bald head, now at his ankles. As the doctor went in, Nikita jumped up from his heap of litter and stood at attention.

"Good-day, Nikita," Andrey Yefimitch said mildly. "That Jew should be provided with boots or something; he will catch cold."

"Certainly, your honor. I'll inform the superintendent."

"Please do; ask him in my name. Tell him that I asked."

The door into the ward was open. Ivan Dmitritch, lying propped on his elbow on the bed, listened in alarm to the unfamiliar voice, and suddenly recognized the doctor. He trembled all over with anger, jumped up, and with a red and wrathful face, with his eyes starting out of his head, ran out into the middle of the road.

"The doctor has come!" he shouted, and broke into a laugh. "At last! Gentlemen, I congratulate you. The doctor is honoring us with a visit! Cursed reptile!" he shrieked, and stamped in a frenzy such as had never been seen in the ward before. "Kill the reptile! No, killing's too good. Drown him in the midden-pit!"

Andrey Yefimitch, hearing this, looked into the ward from the entry and asked gently: "What for?"

"What for?" shouted Ivan Dmitritch, going up to him with a menacing air and convulsively wrapping himself in his dressing-gown. "What for? Thief!" he said with a look of repulsion, moving his lips as though he would spit at him. "Quack! Hangman!"

"Calm yourself," said Andrey Yefimitch, smiling guiltily. "I assure you I have never stolen anything; and as to the rest, most likely you greatly exaggerate. I see you are angry with me. Calm yourself, I beg, if you can, and tell me coolly what are you angry for?"

"What are you keeping me here for?"

"Because you are ill."

"Yes, I am ill. But you know dozens, hundreds of madmen are walking about in freedom because your ignorance is incapable of distinguishing them from the sane. Why am I and these poor wretches to be shut up here like scapegoats for all the rest? You, your assistant, the superintendent, and all your hospital rabble, are immeasurably inferior to every one of us morally; why then are we shut up and you not? Where's the logic of it?"

"Morality and logic don't come in, it all depends on chance. If anyone is shut up he has to stay, and if anyone is not shut up he can walk about, that's all. There is neither morality nor logic in my being a doctor and your being a mental patient, there is nothing but idle chance."

"That twaddle I don't understand. . . ." Ivan Dmitritch brought out in a hollow voice, and he sat down on his bed.

Moiseika, whom Nikita did not venture to search in the presence of the doctor, laid out on his bed pieces of bread, bits of paper, and little bones, and, still shivering with cold, began rapidly in a singsong voice saying something in Yiddish. He most likely imagined that he had opened a shop.

"Let me out," said Ivan Dmitritch, and his voice quivered.

"I cannot."

"But why, why?"

"Because it is not in my power. Think, what use will it be to you if I do let you out? Go. The towns-people or the police will detain you or bring you back."

"Yes, yes, that's true," said Ivan Dmitritch, and he rubbed his forehead. "It's awful! But what am I to do, what?"

Andrey Yefimitch liked Ivan Dmitritch's voice and his intelligent young face with its grimaces. He longed to be kind to the young man and soothe him; he sat down on the bed beside him, thought, and said:

"You ask me what to do. The very best thing in your position would be to run away. But, unhappily, that is useless. You would be taken up. When society protects itself from the criminal, mentally deranged, or otherwise inconvenient people, it is invincible. There is only one thing left for you: to resign yourself to the thought that your presence here is inevitable."

"It is no use to anyone."

"So long as prisons and madhouses exist someone must be shut up in them. If not you, I. If not I, some third person. Wait till in the distant future prisons and madhouses no longer exist, and there will be neither bars on the windows nor hospital gowns. Of course, that time will come sooner or later."

Ivan Dmitritch smiled ironically.

"You are jesting," he said, screwing up his eyes. "Such gentlemen as you and your assistant Nikita have nothing to do with the future, but you may be sure, sir, better days will come! I may express myself cheaply, you may laugh, but the dawn of a new life is at hand; truth and justice will triumph, and—our turn will come! I shall not live to see it, I shall perish, but some people's great-grandsons will see it. I greet them with all my heart and rejoice with them! Onward! God be your help, friends!"

With shining eyes Ivan Dmitritch got up, and stretching his hands towards the window, went on with emotion in his voice:

"From behind these bars I bless you! Hurrah for truth and justice! I rejoice!"

"I see no particular reason to rejoice," said Andrey Yefimitch, who thought Ivan Dmitritch's movement theatrical, though he was delighted by it. "Prisons and madhouses there will not be, and truth, as you have just expressed it, will triumph; but the reality of things, you know, will not change, the laws of nature will still remain the same. People will suffer pain, grow old, and die just as they do now.

However magnificent a dawn lighted up your life, you would yet in the end be nailed up in a coffin and thrown into a hole."

"And immortality?"

"Oh, come, now!"

"You don't believe in it, but I do. Somebody in Dostoevsky or Voltaire said that if there had not been a God, men would have invented him. And I firmly believe that if there is no immortality the great intellect of man will sooner or later invent it."

"Well said," observed Andrey Yefimitch, smiling with pleasure; "it's a good thing you have faith. With such a belief one may live happily even shut up within walls. You have studied somewhere, I presume?"

"Yes, I have been at the university, but did not complete my studies."

"You are a reflecting and a thoughtful man. In any surroundings you can find tranquility in yourself. Free and deep thinking which strives for the comprehension of life, complete contempt for the foolish bustle of the world—those are two blessings beyond any that man has ever known. And you can possess them even though you lived behind threefold bars. Diogenes lived in a tub, yet he was happier than all the kings of the earth."

"Your Diogenes was a blockhead," said Ivan Dmitritch morosely. "Why do you talk to me about Diogenes and some foolish comprehension of life?" he cried, growing suddenly angry and leaping up. "I love life; I love it passionately. I have the mania of persecution, a continual agonizing terror; but I have moments when I am overwhelmed by the thirst for life, and then I am afraid of going mad. I want dreadfully to live, dreadfully!"

He walked up and down the ward in agitation, and said, dropping his voice:

"When I dream I am haunted by phantoms. People come to me, I hear voices and music, and I fancy I am walking through woods or by the seashore, and I long so passionately for movement, for interests. Come, tell me, what news is there?" asked Ivan Dmitritch; "what's happening?"

"Do you wish to know about the town or in general?"

"Well, tell me first about the town, and then in general."

"Well, in the town it is appallingly dull. There's no one to say a word to, no one to listen to. There are no new people. A young doctor called Hobotov has come here recently."

"He had come in my time. Well, he is a low cad, isn't he?"

"Yes, he is a man of no culture. It's strange, you know. Judging by every sign, there is no intellectual stagnation in our capital cities; there is a movement—so there must be real people there too; but for some reason they always send us such men as I would rather not see. It's an unlucky town!"

"Yes, it is an unlucky town," sighed Ivan Dmitritch, and he laughed. "And how are things in general? What are they writing in the papers and reviews?"

It was by now dark in the ward. The doctor got up, and, standing, began to describe what was being written abroad and in Russia, and the tendency of thought that could be noticed now. Ivan Dmitritch listened attentively and put questions, but suddenly, as though recalling something terrible, clutched at his head and lay down on the bed with his back to the doctor.

"What's the matter?" asked Andrey Yefimitch.

"You will not hear another word from me," said Ivan Dmitritch rudely. "Leave me alone."

"Why so?"

"I tell you, leave me alone. Why the devil do you persist?"

Andrey Yefimitch shrugged his shoulders, heaved a sigh, and went out. As he crossed the entry he said: "You might clear up here, Nikita . . . there's an awfully stuffy smell."

"Certainly, your honor."

"What an agreeable young man!" thought Andrey Yefimitch, going back to his flat. "In all the years I have been living here I do believe he is the first I have met with whom one can talk. He is capable of reasoning and is interested in just the right things."

While he was reading, and afterwards, while he was going to bed, he kept thinking about Ivan Dmitritch, and when he woke next morning he remembered that he had the day before made the acquaintance of an intelligent and interesting man, and determined to visit him again as soon as possible.

X

Ivan Dmitritch was lying in the same position as on the previous day, with his head clutched in both hands and his legs drawn up. His face was not visible.

"Good day, my friend," said Andrey Yefimitch. "You are not asleep, are you?"

"In the first place, I am not your friend," Ivan Dmitritch articulated into the pillow; "and in the second, your efforts are useless; you will not get one word out of me."

"Strange," muttered Andrey Yefimitch in confusion. "Yesterday we talked peacefully, but suddenly for some reason you took offence and broke off all at once. Probably I expressed myself awkwardly, or perhaps gave utterance to some idea that did not fit in with your convictions."

"Yes, a likely idea!" said Ivan Dmitritch, sitting up and looking at the doctor with irony and uneasiness. His eyes were red. "You can go and spy and probe somewhere else, it's no use your doing it here. I knew yesterday what you had come for."

"A strange fancy," laughed the doctor. "So you suppose me to be a spy?

"Yes, I do. A spy or a doctor who has been charged to test me—it's all the same—"

"Oh, excuse me, what a queer fellow you are really!"

The doctor sat down on the stool near the bed and shook his head reproachfully.

"But let us suppose you are right," he said, "let us suppose that I am treacherously trying to trap you into saying something so as to betray you to the police. You would be arrested and then tried. But would you be any worse off being tried and in prison than you are here? If you are banished to a settlement, or even sent to penal servitude, would it be worse than being shut up in this ward? I imagine it would be no worse. What, then, are you afraid of?"

These words evidently had an effect on Ivan Dmitritch. He sat down quietly.

It was between four and five in the afternoon—the time when Andrey Yefimitch usually walked up and down his rooms, and Daryushka asked whether it was not time for his beer. It was a still, bright day.

"I came out for a walk after dinner, and here I have come, as you see," said the doctor. "It is quite spring."

"What month is it? March?" asked Ivan Dmitritch.

"Yes, the end of March."

"Is it very muddy?"

"No, not very. There are already paths in the garden."

"It would be nice now to drive in an open carriage somewhere into the country," said Ivan Dmitritch, rubbing his red eyes as though he were just awake, "then to come home to a warm, snug study, and . . . and to have a decent doctor to cure one's headache. It's so long since I have lived like a human being. It's disgusting here! Insufferably disgusting!"

After his excitement of the previous day he was exhausted and listless, and spoke unwillingly. His fingers twitched, and from his face it could be seen that he had a splitting headache.

"There is no real difference between a warm, snug study and this ward," said Andrey Yefimitch. "A man's peace and contentment do not lie outside a man, but in himself."

"What do you mean?"

"The ordinary man looks for good and evil in external things—that is, in carriages, in studies—but a thinking man looks for it in himself."

"You should go and preach that philosophy in Greece, where it's warm and fragrant with the scent of pomegranates, but here it is not suited to the climate. With whom was it I was talking of Diogenes? Was it with you?"

"Yes, with me yesterday."

"Diogenes did not need a study or a warm habitation; it's hot there without. You can lie in your tub and eat oranges and olives. But bring him to Russia to live: he'd be begging to be let indoors in May, let alone December. He'd be doubled up with the cold."

"No. One can be insensible to cold as to every other pain. Marcus Aurelius says: 'A pain is a vivid idea of pain; make an effort of will to change that idea, dismiss it, cease to complain, and the pain will disappear.' That is true. The wise man, or simply the reflecting, thoughtful man, is distinguished precisely by his contempt for suffering; he is always contented and surprised at nothing."

"Then I am an idiot, since I suffer and am discontented and surprised at the baseness of mankind."

"You are wrong in that; if you will reflect more on the subject you will understand how insignificant is all that external world that agitates us. One must strive for the comprehension of life, and in that is true happiness."

"Comprehension . . ." repeated Ivan Dmitritch frowning. "External, internal. Excuse me, but I don't understand it. I only know," he said, getting up and looking angrily at the doctor—"I only know that God has created me of warm blood and nerves, yes, indeed! If organic tissue is capable of life it must react to every stimulus. And I do! To pain I respond with tears and outcries, to baseness with indignation, to filth with loathing. To my mind, that is just what is called life. The lower the organism, the less sensitive it is, and the more feebly it reacts to stimulus; and the higher it is, the more responsively and vigorously it reacts to reality. How is it you don't know that? A doctor, and not know such trifles! To despise suffering, to be always contented, and to be surprised at nothing, one must reach this condition"—and Ivan Dmitritch pointed to the peasant who was a mass of fat—"or to harden oneself by suffering to such a point that one loses all sensibility to it—that is, in other words, to cease to live. You must excuse me, I am not a sage or a philosopher," Ivan Dmitritch continued with irritation, "and I don't understand anything about it. I am not capable of reasoning."

"On the contrary, your reasoning is excellent."

"The Stoics, whom you are parodying, were remarkable people, but their doctrine crystallized two thousand years ago and has not advanced, and will not advance, an inch forward, since it is not practical or living. It had a success only with the minority, which spends its life in savoring all sorts of theories and ruminating over them; the majority did not understand it. A doctrine which advocates indifference to wealth and to the comforts of life, and a contempt for suffering and death, is quite unintelligible to the vast majority of men, since that majority has never known wealth or the comforts of life; and to despise suffering would mean to it despising life itself, since the whole existence of man is made up of the sensations of hunger, cold, injury, loss, and a Hamlet-like dread of death. The whole of life lies in these sensations; one may be oppressed by it, one may hate it, but one cannot despise it. Yes, so, I repeat, the doctrine of the Stoics can never have a future; from the beginning of time up to today you see continually increasing the struggle, the sensibility to pain, the capacity of responding to stimulus."

Ivan Dmitritch suddenly lost the thread of his thoughts, stopped, and rubbed his forehead with vexation.

"I meant to say something important, but I have lost it," he said. "What was I saying?" Oh, yes! This is what I mean: one of the Stoics sold himself into slavery to redeem his neighbor, so, you see, even a Stoic did react to stimulus, since, for such a generous act as the destruction of oneself for the sake of one's neighbor, he must have had a soul capable of pity and indignation. Here in prison I have forgotten everything I have learned, or else I could have recalled something else. Take Christ, for instance: Christ responded to reality by weeping, smiling, being sorrowful and moved to wrath, even overcome by misery. He did not go to meet His sufferings with a smile, He did not despise death, but prayed in the Garden of Gethsemane that this cup might pass Him by."

Ivan Dmitritch laughed and sat down.

"Granted that a man's peace and contentment lie not outside but in himself," he said, "granted that one must despise suffering and not be surprised at anything, yet on what ground do you preach the theory? Are you a sage? A philosopher?"

"No, I am not a philosopher, but everyone ought to preach it because it is reasonable."

"No, I want to know how it is that you consider yourself competent to judge of 'comprehension,' contempt for suffering, and so on. Have you ever suffered? Have you any idea of suffering? Allow me to ask you, were you ever thrashed in your childhood?"

"No, my parents had an aversion for corporal punishment."

"My father used to flog me cruelly; my father was a harsh, sickly Government clerk with a long nose and a yellow neck. But let us talk of you. No one has laid a finger on you all your life, no one has scared you nor beaten you; you are as strong as a bull. You grew up under your father's wing and studied at his expense, and then you dropped at once into a sinecure. For more than twenty years you have lived rent free with heating, lighting, and service all provided, and had the right to work how you pleased and as much as you pleased, even to do nothing. You were naturally a flabby, lazy man, and so you have tried to arrange your life so that nothing should disturb you or make you move. You have handed over your work to the assistant and the rest of the rabble while you sit in peace and warmth, save money, read, amuse yourself with reflections, with all sorts of lofty nonsense, and" (Ivan Dmitritch looked at the doctor's red nose) "with boozing; in fact, you have seen nothing of life, you know absolutely nothing of it, and are only theoretically acquainted with reality; you despise suffering and are surprised at nothing for a very simple reason: vanity of vanities, the external and the internal, contempt for life, for suffering and for death, comprehension, true happiness—that's the philosophy that suits the Russian sluggard best. You see a peasant beating his wife, for instance. Why interfere? Let him beat her, they will both die sooner or later, anyway; and, besides, he who beats injures by his blows, not the person he is beating, but himself. To get drunk is stupid and unseemly, but if you drink you die, and if you don't drink you die. A peasant woman comes with toothache . . . well, what of it? Pain is the idea of pain, and besides 'there is no living in this world without illness; we shall all die, and so, go away, woman, don't hinder me from thinking and drinking vodka.' A young man asks advice, what he is to do, how he is to live; anyone else would think before answering, but you have got the answer ready: strive for 'comprehension' or for true happiness. And what is that fantastic 'true happiness'? There's no answer, of course. We are kept here behind barred windows, tortured, left to rot; but that is very good and reasonable, because there is no difference at all between this ward and a warm, snug study. A convenient philosophy. You can do nothing, and your conscience is clear, and you feel you are wise. No, sir, it is not philosophy, it's not thinking, it's not breadth of vision, but laziness, fakirism, drowsy stupefaction. "Yes," cried Ivan Dmitritch, getting angry again, "you despise suffering, but I'll be bound if you pinch your finger in the door you will howl at the top of your voice."

"And perhaps I shouldn't howl," said Andrey Yefimitch, with a gentle smile.

"Oh, I dare say! Well, if you had a stroke of paralysis, or supposing some fool or bully took advantage of his position and rank to insult you in public, and if you knew he could do it with impurity, then you would understand what it means to put people off with comprehension and true happiness."

"That's original," said Andrey Yefimitch, laughing with pleasure and rubbing his hands. "I am agreeably struck by your inclination for drawing generalizations, and the sketch of my character you have just drawn is simply brilliant. I must confess that talking to you gives me great pleasure. Well, I've listened to you, and now you must graciously listen to me."

XI

The conversation went on for about an hour longer, and apparently made a deep impression on Andrey Yefimitch. He began going to the ward every day. He went there in the mornings and after dinner, and often the dusk of evening found him in conversation with Ivan Dmitritch. At first Ivan Dmitritch held aloof from him, suspected him of evil designs, and openly expressed his hostility. But afterwards, he got used to him, and his abrupt manner changed to one of condescending irony.

Soon it was all over the hospital that the doctor, Andrey Yefimitch, had taken to visiting Ward No. 6. No one—neither Sergey Sergeyitch, nor Nikita, nor the nurses—could conceive why he went there, why he stayed there for hours together, what he was talking about, and why he did not write prescriptions. His actions seemed strange. Often Mihail Averyanitch did not find him at home, which had never happened in the past, and Daryushka was greatly perturbed, for the doctor drank his beer now at no definite time, and sometimes was even late for dinner.

One day—it was at the end of June—Dr. Hobotov went to see Andrey Yefimitch about something. Not finding him at home, he proceeded to look for him in the yard; there he was told that the old doctor had gone to see the mental patients. Going into the lodge and stopping in the entry, Hobotov heard the following conversation:

"We shall never agree, and you will not succeed in converting me to your faith," Ivan Dmitritch was saying irritably; "you are utterly ignorant of reality, and you have never known suffering, but have only like a leech fed beside the sufferings of others, while I have been in continual suffering from the day of my birth till today. For that reason, I tell you frankly, I consider myself superior to you and more competent in every respect. It's not for you to teach me."

"I have absolutely no ambition to convert you to my faith," said Andrey Yefimetch gently, and with regret that others refused to understand him. "And that is not what matters, my friend; what matters is not that you have suffered and I have not. Joy and suffering are passing; let us leave them, never mind them. What matters is that you and I think; we see in each other people who are capable of thinking and reasoning, and that is a common bond between us however different our views. If you knew, my friend, how sick I am of the universal senselessness, ineptitude, stupidity, and with what delight I always talk with you! You are an intelligent man, and I enjoy your company."

Hobotov opened the door an inch and glanced into the ward; Ivan Dmitritch in his night cap and the doctor Andrey Yefimitch were sitting side by side on the bed. The madman was grimacing, twitching, and convulsively wrapping himself in his gown, while the doctor sat motionless with bowed head, and his face was red and looked helpless and sorrowful. Hobotov shrugged his shoulders, grinned, and glanced at Nikita. Nikita shrugged his shoulders too.

Next day Hobotov went to the lodge, accompanied by the assistant. Both stood in the entry and listened.

"I fancy our old man has gone clean off his chump!" said Hobotov as he came out of the lodge.

"Lord have mercy upon us sinners!" sighed the decorous Sergey Sergeyitch, scrupulously avoiding the puddles that he might not muddy his polished boots. "I must own, honored Yevgeny Fyodoritch, I have been expecting it for a long time."

XII

After this Andrey Yefimitch began to notice a mysterious air in all around him. The attendants, the nurses, and the patients looked at him inquisitively when they met him, and then whispered together. The superintendent's little daughter Masha, whom he liked to meet in the hospital garden, for some reason ran away from him now when he went up with a smile to stroke her on the head. The postmaster no longer said "perfectly true," as he listened to him, but in accountable confusion muttered, "Yes, yes, yes," and looked at him with a grieved and thoughtful expression; for some reason he took to advising his friend to give up vodka and beer, but as a man of delicate feeling he did not say this directly, but hinted it, telling him first about the commanding officer of his battalion, an excellent man, and then about the priest of the regiment, a capital fellow, both of whom drank and fell ill, but on giving up drinking completely regained their health. On two or three occasions Andrey Yefimitch was visited by his colleague Hobotov, who also advised him to give up spirituous liquors, and for no apparent reason recommended him to take bromide.

In August Andrey Yefimitch got a letter from the mayor of the town asking him to come on very important business. On arriving at the town hall at the time fixed, Andrey Yefimitch found there the military commander, the superintendent of the district school, a member of the town council, Hobotov, and a plump, fair gentleman who was introduced to him as a doctor. This doctor, with a Polish surname difficult to pronounce, lived at a pedigree stud farm twenty miles away, and was now on a visit to the town.

"There's something that concerns you," said the member of the town council, addressing Andrey Yefimitch after they had all greeted one another and sat down to the table. "Here Yevgeny Fyodoritch says that there is not room for the dispensary in the main building, and that it ought to be transferred to one of the lodges. That's of no consequence—of course it can be transferred, but the point is that the lodge wants doing up."

"Yes, it would have to be done up," said Andrey Yefimitch after a moment's thought. "If the corner lodge, for instance, were fitted up as a dispensary, I imagine it would cost at least five hundred rubles. An unproductive expenditure!"

Everyone was silent for a space.

"I had the honor of submitting to you ten years ago," Andrey Yefimitch went on in a low voice, "that the hospital in its present form is a luxury for the town beyond its means. It was built in the forties, but things were different then. The town spends too much on unnecessary buildings and superfluous staff. I believe with a different system two model hospitals might be maintained for the same money."

"Well, let us have a different system, then!" the member of the town council said briskly.

"I have already had the honor of submitting to you that the medical department should be transferred to the supervision of the Zemstvo."

"Yes, transfer the money to the Zemstvo and they will steal it," laughed the fair-haired doctor.

"That's what it always comes to," the member of the council assented, and he also laughed.

Andrey Yefimitch looked with apathetic, lusterless eyes at the fair-haired doctor and said: "One should be just."

Again there was silence. Tea was brought in. The military commander, for some reason much embarrassed, touched Andrey Yefimitch's hand across the table and said: "You have quite forgotten us, doctor. But of course you are a hermit: you don't play cards and don't like women. You would be dull with fellows like us."

They all began saying how boring it was for a decent person to live in such a town. No theatre, no music, and at the last dance at the club there had been about twenty ladies and only two gentlemen. The young men did not dance, but spent all the time crowding round the refreshment bar or playing cards.

Not looking at anyone and speaking slowly in a low voice, Andrey Yefimitch began saying what a pity, what a terrible pity it was that the towns-people should waste their vital energy, their hearts, and their minds on cards and gossip, and should have neither the power nor the inclination to spend their time in interesting conversation and reading, and should refuse to take advantage of the enjoyments of the mind. The mind alone was interesting and worthy of attention; all the rest was low and petty. Hobotov listened to his colleague attentively and suddenly asked:

"Andrey Yefimitch, what day of the month is it?"

Having received an answer, the fair-haired doctor and he, in the tone of examiners conscious of their lack of skill, began asking Andrey Yefimitch what was the day of the week, how many days there were in the year, and whether it was true that there was a remarkable prophet living in Ward No. 6.

In response to the last question Andrey Yefimitch turned rather red and said: "Yes, he is mentally deranged, but he is an interesting young man."

They asked him no other questions.

When he was putting on his overcoat in the entry the military commander laid a hand on his shoulder and said with a sigh:

"It's time for us old fellows to rest!"

As he came out of the hall, Andrey Yefimitch understood that it had been a committee appointed to inquire into his mental condition. He recalled the questions that had been asked him, flushed crimson, and for some reason, for the first time in his life, felt bitterly grieved for medical science.

"My God," he thought, remembering how these doctors had just examined him; "why, they have only lately been hearing lectures on mental pathology; they had passed an examination—what's the explanation of this crass ignorance? They have not a conception of mental pathology!"

And for the first time in his life he felt insulted and moved to anger.

In the evening of the same day Mihail Averyanitch came to see him. The postmaster went up to him without waiting to greet him, took him by both hands, and said in an agitated voice:

"My dear fellow, my dear friend, show me that you believe in my genuine affection and look on me as your friend!" And preventing Andrey Yefimitch from speaking, he went on, growing excited: "I love you for your culture and nobility of soul. Listen to me, my dear fellow. The rules of their profession compel the doctors to conceal the truth from you, but I blurt out the plain truth like a soldier. You are not well! Excuse me, my dear fellow, but it is the truth; everyone about you has been noticing it for a long time. Dr. Yevgeny Fyodoritch has just told me that it is essential for you to rest and distract your mind for the sake of your health. Perfectly true! Excellent! In a day or two I am taking a holiday and am going away for a sniff of a different atmosphere. Show that you are a friend to me; let us go together! Let us go for a jaunt as in the good old days."

"I feel perfectly well," said Andrey Yefimitch after a moment's thought. "I can't go away. Allow me to show you my friendship in some other way."

To go off with no object, without his books, without his Daryushka, without his beer, to break abruptly through the routine of life, established for twenty years—the idea for the first minute struck him as wild and fantastic, but he remembered the conversation at the Zemstvo committee and the depressing feelings with which he had returned home, and the thought of a brief absence from the town in which stupid people looked on him as a madman was pleasant to him.

"And where precisely do you intend to go?" he asked.

"To Moscow, to Petersburg, to Warsaw. I spent the five happiest years of my life in Warsaw. What a marvelous town! Let us go, my dear fellow!"

XIII

A week later it was suggested to Andrey Yefimitch that he should have a rest—that is, send in his resignation—a suggestion he received with indifference; a week later still, Mihail Averyanitch and he were sitting in a posting carriage driving to the nearest railway station. The days were cool and bright, with a blue sky and a transparent distance. They were two days driving the hundred and fifty miles to the railway station, and stayed two nights on the way. When at the posting station the glasses given them for their tea had not been properly washed, or the drivers were slow in harnessing the horses, Mihail Averyanitch would turn crimson, and quivering all over would shout:

"Hold your tongue! Don't argue!"

And in the carriage he talked without ceasing for a moment, describing his campaigns in the Caucasus and in Poland. What adventures he had had, what meetings! He talked loudly and opened his eyes so wide with wonder that he might well be thought to be lying. Moreover, as he talked he breathed in Andrey Yefimitch's face and laughed into his ear. This bothered the doctor and prevented him from thinking or concentrating his mind.

In the train they traveled, from motives of economy, third-class in a non-smoking compartment. Half the passengers were decent people. Mihail Averyanitch soon made friends with everyone, and moving from one seat to another, kept saying loudly that they ought not to travel by these appalling lines. It was a regular swindle! A very different thing riding on a good horse: one could do over seventy miles a day and feel fresh and well after it. And our bad harvests were due to the draining of Pinsk marshes; altogether, the way things were done was dreadful. He got excited, talked loudly, and would not let others peak. This endless chatter to the accompaniment of loud laughter and expressive gestures wearied Andrey Yefimitch.

"Which of us is the madman?" he thought with vexation. "I, who try not to disturb my fellow passengers in any way, or this egoist who thinks that he is cleverer and more interesting than anyone here, and so will leave no one in peace?"

In Moscow Mihail Averyanitch put on a military coat without epaulettes and trousers with red braid on them. He wore a military cap and overcoat in the street, and soldiers saluted him. It seemed to Andrey Yefimitch, now, that his companion was a man who had flung away all that was good and kept only what was bad of all the characteristics of a country gentleman that he had once possessed. He liked to be waited on even when it was quite unnecessary. The matches would be lying before him on the table, and he would see them and shout to the waiter to give him the matches; he did not hesitate to appear before a maidservant in nothing but his underclothes; he used the familiar mode of address to all footmen indiscriminately, even old men, and when he was angry called them fools and blockheads. This, Andrey Yefimitch thought, was like a gentleman, but disgusting.

First of all Mihail Averyanitch led his friend to the Iversky Madonna. He prayed fervently, shedding tears and bowing down to the earth, and when he had finished, heaved a deep sigh and said:

"Even though one does not believe it makes one somehow easier when one prays a little. Kiss the icon, my dear fellow."

Andrey Yefimitch was embarrassed and he kissed the image, while Mihail Averyanitch pursed up his lips and prayed in a whisper, and again tears came into his eyes. Then they went to the Kremlin and looked there at the Tsar-cannon and the Tsar-bell, and even touched them with their fingers, admired the view over the river, visited St. Savior's and the Rumyantsev museum.

They dined at Tyestov's. Mihail Averyanitch looked a long time at the menu, stroking his whiskers, and said in the tone of a gourmand accustomed to dine in restaurants:

"We shall see what you give us to eat today, angel!"

XIV

The doctor walked about, looked at things, ate and drank, but he had all the while one feeling: annoyance with Mihail Averyanitch. He longed to have a rest from his friend, to get away from him, to hide himself, while the friend thought it his duty not to let the doctor move a step away from him, and to provide him with as many distractions as possible. When there was nothing to look at he entertained him with conversation. For two days Andrey Yefimitch endured it, but on the third he announced to his friend that he was ill and wanted to stay at home for the whole day; his friend replied that in that case he would stay too—that really he needed rest, for he was run off his legs already. Andrey Yefimitch lay on the sofa, with his face to the back, and clenching his teeth, listened to his friend, who assured him with heat that sooner or later France would certainly thrash Germany, that there were a great many scoundrels in Moscow, and that it was impossible to judge of a horse's quality by its outward appearance. The doctor began to have a buzzing in his ears and palpitations of the heart, but out of delicacy could not bring himself to beg his friend to go away or hold his tongue. Fortunately, Mihail Averyanitch grew weary of sitting in the hotel room, and after dinner he went out for a walk.

As soon as he was alone, Andrey Yefimitch abandoned himself to a feeling of relief. How pleasant to lie motionless on the sofa and to know that one is alone in the room! Real happiness is impossible without solitude. The fallen angel betrayed God probably because he longed for solitude, of which the angels know nothing. Andrey Yefimitch wanted to think about what he had seen and heard during the last few days, but he could not get Mihail Averyanitch out of his head.

"Why, he has taken a holiday and come with me out of friendship, out of generosity," thought the doctor with vexation; "nothing could be worse than this friendly supervision. I suppose he is good-natured and generous and a lively fellow, but he is a bore. An insufferable bore. In the same way there are people who never say anything but what is clever and good, yet one feels that they are dull-witted people."

For the following days Andrey Yefimitch declared himself ill and would not leave the hotel room; he lay with his face to the back of the sofa, and suffered agonies of weariness when his friend entertained him with conversation, or rested when his friend was absent. He was vexed with himself for having come, and with his friend, who grew every day more talkative and more free and easy; he could not succeed in attuning his thoughts to a serious and lofty level.

"This is what I get from the real life Ivan Dmitritch talked about," he thought, angry at his own pettiness. "It's of no consequence, though. I shall go home, and everything will go on as before."

It was the same thing in Petersburg too; for whole days together he did not leave the hotel room, but lay on the sofa and only got up to drink beer.

Mihail Averyanitch was all haste to get to Warsaw.

"My dear man, what should I go there for?" said Andrey Yefimitch in an imploring voice. "You go alone and let me get home! I entreat you!"

"On no account," protested Mihail Averyanitch. "It's a marvelous town."

Andrey Yefimitch had not the strength of will to insist on his own way, and much against his inclination went to Warsaw. There he did not leave the hotel room, but lay on the sofa, furious with himself, with his friend, and with the waiters, who obstinately refused to understand Russian; while Mihail Averyanitch, healthy, hearty, and full of spirits as usual, went about the town from morning to night, looking for his old acquaintances. Several times he did not return home at night. After one night spent in some unknown haunt he returned home early in the morning, in a violently excited condition, with a red face and tousled hair. For a long time he walked up and down the rooms muttering something to himself, then stopped and said:

"Honor before everything."

After walking up and down a little longer he clutched his head in both hands and pronounced in a tragic voice: "Yes, honor before everything! Accursed be the moment when the idea first entered my head to visit this Babylon! My dear friend," he added, addressing the doctor, "you may despise me, I have played and lost; lend me five hundred rubles!"

Andrey Yefimitch counted out five hundred rubles and gave them to his friend without a word. The latter, still crimson with shame and anger incoherently articulated some useless vow, put on his cap, and went out. Returning two hours later he flopped into an easy-chair, heaved a loud sigh, and said:

"My honor is saved. Let us go, my friend; I do not care to remain another hour in this accursed town. Scoundrels! Austrian spies!"

By the time the friends were back in their own town it was November, and deep snow was lying in the streets. Dr. Hobotov had Andrey Yefimitch's post; he was still living in his old lodgings, waiting for Andrey Yefimitch to arrive and clear out of the hospital apartments. The plain woman whom he called his cook was already established in one of the lodges.

Fresh scandals about the hospital were going the round of the town. It was said that the plain woman had quarreled with the superintendent, and that the latter had crawled on his knees before her begging forgiveness. On the very first day he arrived Andrey Yefimitch had to look out for lodgings.

"My friend," the postmaster said to him timidly "excuse an indiscreet question: what means have you at your disposal?"

Andrey Yefimitch, without a word, counted out his money and said: "Eighty-six rubles."

"I don't mean that," Mihail Averyanitch brought out in confusion, misunderstanding him; "I mean, what have you to live on?"

"I tell you, eighty-six rubles. I have nothing else."

Mihail Averyanitch looked upon the doctor as an honorable man, yet he suspected that he had accumulated a fortune of at least twenty thousand. Now learning that Andrey Yefimitch was a beggar, that he had nothing to live on, he was for some reason suddenly moved to tears and embraced his friend.

XV

Andrey Yefimitch now lodged in a little house with three windows. There were only three rooms besides the kitchen in the little house. The doctor lived in two of them, which looked into the street, while Daryushka and the landlady with her three children lived in the third room and the kitchen. Sometimes the landlady's lover, a drunken peasant who was rowdy and reduced the children and Daryushka to terror, would come for the night. When he arrived and established himself in the kitchen and demanded vodka, they all felt very uncomfortable, and the doctor would be moved by pity to take the crying children into his room and let them lie on his floor, and this gave him great satisfaction.

He got up as before at eight o'clock, and after his morning tea sat down to read his old books and magazines: he had no money for new ones. Either because the books were old, or perhaps because of the change in his surroundings, reading exhausted him, and did not grip his attention as before. That he might not spend his time in idleness he made a detailed catalogue of his books and gummed little labels on their backs, and this mechanical, tedious work seemed to him more interesting than reading. The monotonous, tedious work lulled his thoughts to sleep in some unaccountable way, and the time passed quickly while he thought of nothing. Even sitting in the kitchen, peeling potatoes with Dar-yushka or picking over the buckwheat grain, seemed to him interesting. On Saturdays and Sundays he went to church. Standing near the wall and half closing his eyes, he listened to the singing and thought of his father, of his mother, of the university, of the religions of the world; he felt calm and melancholy, and as he went out of the church afterwards he regretted that the service was so soon over. He went twice to the hospital to talk to Ivan Dmitritch. But on both occasions Ivan Dmitritch was unusually excited and ill-humored; he bade the doctor leave him in peace, as he had long been sick of empty chatter, and declared, to make up for all his sufferings, he asked from the damned scoundrels only one favor—solitary confinement. Surely they would not refuse him even that? On both occasions when Andrey Yefimitch was taking leave of him and wishing him good-night, he answered rudely and said:

"Go to hell!"

And Andrey Yefimitch did not know now whether to go to him for the third time or not. He longed to go.

In old days, Andrey Yefimitch used to walk about his rooms and think in the interval after dinner, but now from dinnertime till evening tea he lay on the sofa with his face to the back and gave himself up to trivial thoughts which he could not struggle against. He was mortified that after more than twenty years of service he had been given neither a pension nor any assistance. It is true that he had not done his work honestly, but, then, all who are in the Service get a pension without distinction whether they are honest or not. Contemporary justice lies precisely in the bestowal of qualities or capacities, but for service whatever it may have been like. Why was he alone to be an exception? He had no money at all. He was ashamed to pass by the shop and look at the woman who owned it. He owed thirty-two rubles for beer already. There was money owing to the landlady also. Daryushka sold old clothes and books on the sly, and told lies to the landlady, saying that the doctor was just going to receive a large sum of money.

He was angry with himself for having wasted on traveling the thousand rubles he had saved up. How useful that thousand rubles would have been now! He was vexed that people would not leave him in peace. Hobotov thought it his duty to look in on his sick colleague from time to time. Everything about him was revolting to Andrey Yefimitch—his well-fed face and vulgar, condescending tone, and his use of the word "colleague," and his high-top boots the most revolting thing was that he thought it was his duty to treat Andrey Yefimitch, and thought that he really was treating him. On every visit he brought a bottle of bromide and rhubarb pills.

Mihail Averyanitch, too, thought it his duty to visit his friend and entertain him. Every time he went in to Andrey Yefimitch with an affectation of ease, laughed constrainedly, and began assuring him that he was looking very well today, and that, thank God, he was on the high road to recovery, and from this it might be concluded that he looked on his friend's condition as hopeless. He had not yet repaid his Warsaw debt, and was overwhelmed by shame; he was constrained, and so tried to laugh louder and talk more amusingly. His anecdotes and descriptions seemed endless now, and were an agony both to Andrey Yefimitch and himself.

In his presence Andrey Yefimitch usually lay on the sofa with his face to the wall, and listened with his teeth clenched; his soul was oppressed with rankling disgust, and after every visit from his friend he felt as though this disgust had risen higher, and was mounting into his throat.

To stifle petty thoughts he made haste to reflect that he himself, and Hobotov, and Mihail Averyanitch would all sooner or later perish without leaving any trace on the world. If one imagined some spirit flying by the earthly globe in space in a million years he would see nothing but clay and bare rocks. Everything—culture and the moral law—would pass away and not even a burdock would grow out of them. Of what consequence was shame in the presence of a shopkeeper, of what consequence was the insignificant Hobotov or the wearisome friendship of Mihail Averyanitch? It was all trivial and nonsensical.

But such reflections did not help him now. Scarcely had he imagined the earthly globe in a million years, when Hobotov in his high-top boots or Mihail Averyanitch with his forced laugh would appear from behind a bare rock, and he even heard the shamefaced whisper: "The Warsaw debt. I will repay it in a day or two, my dear fellow, without fail."

XVI

One day Mihail Averyanitch came after dinner when Yefimitch was lying on the sofa. It so happened that Hobotov arrived at the same time with his bromide. Andrey Yefimitch got up heavily and sat down, leaning both arms on the sofa.

"You have a much better color today than you had yesterday, my dear man," began Mihail Averyanitch. "Yes, you look jolly. Upon my soul, you do!"

"It's high time you were well, colleague," said Hobotov, yawning. "I'll be bound, you are sick of this bobbery."

"And we shall recover," said Mihail Averyanitch cheerfully. "We shall live another hundred years! To be sure!"

"Not a hundred years, but another twenty," Hobotov said reassuringly. "It's all right, all right, colleague; don't lose heart. Don't go piling it on!"

"We'll show what we can do," laughed Mihail Averyanitch, and he slapped his friend on the knee. "We'll show them yet! Next summer, please God, we shall be off to the Caucasus and we will ride all over it on horseback—trot, trot, trot! And when we are back from the Caucasus I shouldn't wonder if we all dance at the wedding." Mihail Averyanitch gave a sly wink. "We'll marry you, my dear boy, we'll marry you."

Andrey Yefimitch felt suddenly that the rising disgust had mounted to his throat; his heart began beating violently.

"That's vulgar," he said, getting up quickly and walking away to the window. "Don't you understand that you are talking vulgar nonsense?"

He meant to go on softly and politely, but against his will he suddenly clenched his fists and raised them above his head.

"Leave me alone," he shouted in a voice unlike his own, flushing crimson and shaking all over. "Go away, both of you!"

Mihail Averyanitch and Hobotov got up and stared at him first with amazement and then with alarm.

"Go away, both!" Andrey Yefimitch went on shouting. "Stupid people! Foolish people! I don't want either your friendship or your medicines, stupid man! Vulgar! Nasty!"

Hobotov and Mihail Averyanitch, looking at each other in bewilderment, staggered to the door and went out. Andrey Yefimitch snatched up the bottle of bromide and flung it after them; the bottle broke with a crash on the door frame.

"Go to the devil!" he shouted in a tearful voice, running out into the passage. "To the devil!"

When his guests were gone Andrey Yefimitch lay down on the sofa, trembling as though in a fever, and went on for a long while repeating: "Stupid people! Foolish people!"

When he was calmer, what occurred to him first of all was the thought that poor Mihail Averyanitch must be feeling fearfully ashamed and depressed now, and that it was all dreadful. Nothing like this had ever happened to him before. Where was his intelligence and his tact? Where was his comprehension of things and his philosophical indifference?

The doctor could not sleep all night for shame and vexation with himself, and at ten o'clock next morning he went to the post office and apologized to the postmaster.

"We won't think again of what has happened," Mihail Averyanitch, greatly touched, said with a sigh, warmly pressing his hand. "Let bygones be bygones. Lyubavkin," he suddenly shouted so loud that all the postmen and other persons present started, "hand a chair; and you wait," he shouted to a peasant woman who was stretching out a registered letter to him through the grating. "Don't you see that I am busy? We will not remember the past," he went on, affectionately addressing Andrey Yefimitch; "sit down, I beg you, my dear fellow."

For a minute he stroked his knees in silence, and then said:

"I have never had a thought of taking offence. Illness is no joke, I understand. Your attack frightened the doctor and me yesterday, and we had a long talk about you afterwards. My dear friend, why won't you treat your illness seriously? You can't go on like this. . . . Excuse me speaking openly as a friend," whispered Mihail Averyanitch. "You live in the most unfavorable surroundings, in a crowd, in uncleanliness, no one to look after you, no money for proper treatment. . . . My dear friend, the doctor and I implore you with all our hearts, listen to our advice: go into the hospital! There you will have wholesome food and attendance and treatment. Though, between ourselves, Yevgeny Fyodoritch is *mauvais ton,* yet he does understand his work; you can fully rely upon him. He has promised me he will look after you."

Andrey Yefimitch was touched by the postmaster's genuine sympathy and the tears, which suddenly glittered on his cheeks.

"My honored friend, don't believe it!" he whispered, laying his hand on his heart; "don't believe them. It's all a sham. My illness is only that in twenty years I have only found one intelligent man in the whole town, and he is mad. I am not ill at all; it's simply that I have got into an enchanted circle which there is no getting out of. I don't care; I am ready for anything."

"Go into the hospital, my dear fellow."

"I don't care if it were into the pit."

"Give me your word, my dear man, that you will obey Yevgeny Fyodoritch in everything."

"Certainly I will give you my word. But I repeat, my honored friend, I have got into an enchanted circle. Now everything, even the genuine sympathy of my friends, leads to the same thing—to my ruin. I am going to my ruin, and I have the manliness to recognize it."

"My dear fellow, you will recover."

"What's the use of saying that?" said Andrey Yefimitch, with irritation. "There are few men who at the end of their lives do not experience what I am experiencing now. When you are told that you have something such as diseased kidneys or enlarged heart, and you begin being treated for it, or are told you are mad or a criminal—that is, in fact, when people suddenly turn their attention to you— you may be sure you have got into an enchanted circle from which you will not escape. You will try to escape and make things worse. You had better give in, for no human efforts can save you. So it seems to me."

Meanwhile the public was crowding at the grating. That he might not be in their way, Andrey Yefimitch got up and began to take leave. Mihail Averyanitch made him promise on his honor once more, and escorted him to the outer door.

Towards evening on the same day Hobotov, in his sheepskin and his high-top boots, suddenly made his appearance, and said to Andrey Yefimitch in a tone as though nothing had happened the day before:

"I have come on business, colleague. I have come to ask you whether you would not join me in a consultation. Eh?"

Thinking that Hobotov wanted to distract his mind with an outing, or perhaps really to enable him to earn something, Andrey Yefimitch put on his coat and hat, and went out with him into the street. He was glad of the opportunity to smooth over his fault of the previous day and to be reconciled, and in his heart thanked Hobotov, who did not even allude to yesterday's scene and was evidently sparing him. One would never have expected such delicacy from this uncultured man.

"Where is your invalid?" asked Andrey Yefimitch.

"In the hospital. I have long waited to show him to you. A very interesting case."

They went into the hospital yard, and going round the main building, turned towards the lodge where the mental cases were kept, and all this, for some reason, in silence. When they went into the lodge Nikita as usual jumped up and stood at attention.

"One of the patients here has a lung complication," Hobotov said in an undertone, going into the ward with Andrey Yefimitch. "You wait here, I'll be back directly. I am going for a stethoscope."

And he went away.

XVII

It was getting dusk. Ivan Dmitritch was lying on his bed with his face thrust into his pillow; the paralytic was sitting motionless, crying quietly and moving his lips. The fat peasant and the former sorter were asleep. It was quiet.

Andrey Yefimitch sat down on Ivan Dmitritch's bed and waited. But half an hour passed, and instead of Hobotov, Nikita came into the ward with a dressing gown, some underlinen, and a pair of slippers in a heap on his arm.

"Please change your things, your honor." He said softly, "Here is your bed; come this way," he added, pointing to an empty bedstead which had obviously been recently brought into the ward. "It's all right; please God, you will recover."

Andrey Yefimitch understood it all. Without saying a word he crossed to the bed to which Nikita pointed and sat down; seeing that Nikita was standing waiting, he undressed entirely and he felt ashamed. Then he put on the hospital clothes; the drawers were very short, the shirt was long, and the dressing gown smelt of smoked fish.

"Please God, you will recover," repeated Nikita, and he gathered up Andrey Yefimitch's clothes into his arms, went out, and shut the door after him.

"No matter . . ." thought Andrey Yefimitch, wrapping himself in his dressing gown in a shame-faced way and feeling that he looked like a convict in his new costume. "It's no matter. It does not matter whether it's a dress-coat or a uniform or this dressing gown."

But, how about his watch? And the notebook that was in the side pocket? And his cigarettes? Where had Nikita taken his clothes? Now perhaps to the day of his death he would not put on trousers, a waistcoat and high boots. It was all somehow strange and even incomprehensible at first. Andrey Yefimitch was even now convinced that there was no difference between his landlady's house and Ward No. 6, that everything in this world was nonsense and vanity of vanities. And yet his hands were trembling, his feet were cold, and he was filled with dread at the thought that soon Ivan Dmitritch would get up and see that he was in a dressing gown. He got up and walked across the room and sat down again.

Here he had been sitting already half an hour, an hour, and he was miserably sick of it: was it really possible to live here a day, a week, and even years like these people? Why, he had been sitting here, had walked about and sat down again; he could get up and look out of window and walk from corner to corner again, and then what? Sit so all the time, like a post, and think? No, that was scarcely possible.

Andrey Yefimitch lay down, but at once got up, wiped the cold sweat from his brow with his sleeve, and felt that his whole face smelt of smoked fish. He walked about again.

"It's some misunderstanding," he said, turning out the palms of his hands in perplexity. "It must be cleared up. There is a misunderstanding."

Meanwhile Ivan Dmitritch woke up; he sat up and propped his cheeks on his fists. He spat. Then he glanced lazily at the doctor, and apparently for the first minute did not understand; but soon his sleepy face grew malicious and mocking.

"Aha! so they have put you in here, too, old fellow?" he said in a voice husky from sleepiness, screwing up one eye. "Very glad to see you. You sucked the blood of others, and now they will suck yours. Excellent!"

"It's a misunderstanding," Andrey Yefimitch brought out, frightened by Ivan Dmitritch's words; he shrugged his shoulders and repeated: "It's some misunderstanding."

Ivan Dmitritch spat again and lay down.

"Cursed life," he grumbled, "and what's bitter and insulting, this life will not end in compensation for our sufferings, it will not end with apotheosis as it would in an opera, but with death; peasants will come and drag one's dead body by the arms and the legs to the cellar. Ugh! Well, it does not matter. We shall have our good time in the other world. I shall come here as a ghost from the other world and frighten these reptiles. I'll turn their hair gray."

Moiseika returned, and, seeing the doctor, held out his hand.

"Give me one little kopeck," he said.

XVIII

Andrey Yefimitch walked away to the window and looked out into the open country. It was getting dark, and on the horizon to the right a cold crimson moon was mounting upwards. Not far from the hospital fence, not much more than two hundred yards away, stood a tall white house shut in by a stone wall. This was the prison.

"So this is real life," thought Andrey Yefimitch and he felt frightened.

The moon and the prison, and the nails on the fence, and the far-away flames at the bone-charring factory were all terrible. Behind him there was the sound of a sigh. Andrey Yefimitch looked round and saw a man with glittering stars and orders on his breast, who was smiling and slyly winking. And this, too, seemed terrible.

Andrey Yefimitch assured himself that there was nothing special about the moon or the prison, that even sane persons wear orders, and that everything in time will decay and turn to earth, but he was suddenly overcome with despair; he clutched at the grating with both hands and shook it with all his might. The strong grating did not yield.

Then that it might not be so dreadful he went to Ivan Dmitritch's bed and sat down.

"I have lost heart, my dear fellow," he muttered, trembling and wiping away the cold sweat, "I have lost heart."

"You should be philosophical," said Ivan Dmitritch ironically.

"My God, my God. Yes, yes. You were pleased to say once that there was no philosophy in Russia, but that all people, even the paltriest, talk philosophy. But you know the philosophizing of the paltriest does not harm anyone," said Andrey Yefimitch in a tone as if he wanted to cry and complain. "Why, then, that malignant laugh, my friend, and how can these paltry creatures help philosophizing if they are not satisfied? For an intelligent, educated man, made in God's image, proud and loving freedom, to have no alternative but to be a doctor in a filthy, stupid, wretched little town, and to spend his whole life among bottles, leeches, mustard plasters! Quackery, narrowness, vulgarity! Oh, my God!"

"You are talking nonsense. If you don't like being a doctor you should have gone in for being a statesman."

"I could not, I could not do anything. We are weak, my dear friend. . . . I used to be indifferent. I reasoned boldly and soundly, but at the first coarse touch of life upon me I have lost heart. . . . Prostration. . . . We are weak, we are poor creatures . . . and you, too, my dear friend, you are intelligent, generous, you drew in good impulses with your mother's milk, but you had hardly entered upon life when you were exhausted and fell ill. . . . Weak, weak!"

Andrey Yefimitch was all the while at the approach of evening tormented by another persistent sensation besides terror and the feeling of resentment. At last he realized that he was longing for a smoke and for beer.

"I am going out, my friend," he said. "I will tell him to bring a light; I can't put up with this. I am not equal to it."

Andrey Yefimitch went to the door and opened it, but at once Nikita jumped up and barred his way.

"Where are you going?" You can't, you can't!" he said. "It's bedtime."

"But I'm only going out for a minute to walk about the yard," said Andrey Yefimitch.

"You can't, you can't; it's forbidden. You know that yourself."

"But what difference will it make to anyone if I do go out?" asked Andrey Yefimitch, shrugging his shoulders. "I don't understand. Nikita, I must go out!" he said in a trembling voice. "I must."

"Don't be disorderly, it's not right," Nikita said peremptorily.

"This is beyond everything," Ivan Dmitritch cried suddenly, and he jumped up. "What right has he not to let you out? How dare they keep us here? I believe it is clearly laid down in the law that no one can be deprived of freedom without trial! It's an outrage! It's tyranny!"

"Of course it's tyranny," said Andrey Yefimitch, encouraged by Ivan Dmitritch's outburst. "I must go out, I want to. He has no right! Open, I tell you."

"Do you hear, you dull-witted brute?" cried Ivan Dmitritch, and he banged on the door with his fist. "Open the door, or I will break it open! Torturer!"

"Open the door," cried Andrey Yefimitch trembling all over; "I insist!"

"Talk away!" Nikita answered through the door, "Talk away."

"Anyhow, go and call Yevgeny Fyodoritch! Say that I beg him to come for a minute!"

"His honor will come of himself tomorrow."

"They will never let us out," Ivan Dmitritch was going on meanwhile. "They will leave us to rot here! Oh, Lord, can there really be no hell in the next world, and will these wretches be forgiven? Where is justice? Open the door, you wretch! I am choking!" he cried in a hoarse voice, and flung himself upon the door. "I'll dash out my brains, murderers!"

Nikita opened the door quickly, and roughly with both his hands and his knee shoved Andrey Yefimitch back, then swung his arm and punched him in the face with his fist. It seemed to Andrey Yefimitch as though a huge salt wave enveloped him from his head downwards and dragged him to the bed; there really was a salt taste in his mouth: most likely the blood was running from his teeth. He waved his arms as though he were trying to swim out and clutched at a bedstead, and at the same moment felt Nikita hit him twice on the back.

Ivan Dmitritch gave a loud scream. He must have been beaten too.

Then all was still, the faint moonlight came through the grating, and a shadow like a net lay on the floor. It was terrible. Andrey Yefimitch lay and held his breath: he was expecting with horror to be struck again. He felt as though someone had taken a sickle, thrust it into him, and turned it round several times in his breast and bowels. He bit the pillow from pain and clenched his teeth, and all at once through the chaos in his brain there flashed the terrible unbearable thought that these people, who seemed now like black shadows in the moonlight, had to endure such pain day by day for years. How could it have happened that for more than twenty years he had not known it and had refused to know it? He knew nothing of pain, had no conception of it, so he was not to blame, but his conscience, as inexorable and as rough as Nikita, made him turn cold from the crown of his head to his heels. He leaped up, tried to cry out with all his might, and to run in haste to kill Nikita, and then Hobotov, the superintendent and the assistant, and then himself; but no sound came from his chest, and his legs would not obey him. Gasping for breath, he tore at the dressing gown and the shirt on his breast, rent them, and fell senseless on the bed.

XIX

Next morning his head ached, there was a droning in his ears and a feeling of utter weakness all over. He was not ashamed at recalling his weakness the day before. He had been cowardly, had even been afraid of the moon, had openly expressed thoughts and feelings such as he had not expected in himself before; for instance, the thought that the paltry people who philosophized were really dissatisfied. But now nothing mattered to him.

He ate nothing; he drank nothing. He lay motionless and silent.

"It is all the same to me," he thought when they asked him questions. "I am not going to answer. It's all the same to me."

After dinner Mihail Averyanitch brought him a quarter of a pound of tea and a pound of fruit pastilles. Daryushka came too and stood for a whole hour by the bed with an expression of dull grief on her face. Dr. Hobotov visited him.

He brought a bottle of bromide and told Nikita to fumigate the ward with something.

Towards evening Andrey Yefimitch died of an apoplectic stroke. At first he had a violent shivering fit and a feeling of sickness; something revolting as it seemed, penetrating through his whole body, even to his finger tips, strained from his stomach to his head and flooded his eyes and ears. There was a greenness before his eyes. Andrey Yefimitch understood that his end had come, and remembered that Ivan Dmitritch, Mihail Averyanitch, and millions of people believed in immortality. And what if it really existed? But he did not want immortality, and he thought of it only for one instant. A herd of deer, extraordinarily beautiful and graceful, of which he had been reading the day before, ran by him; then a peasant woman stretched out her hand to him with a registered letter. Mihail Averyanitch said something, then it all vanished, and Andrey Yefimitch sank into oblivion forever.

The hospital porters came, took him by his arms and his legs, and carried him away to the chapel.

There he lay on the table, with open eyes, and the moon shed its light upon him at night. In the morning Sergey Sergeyitch came, prayed piously before the crucifix, and closed his former chief's eyes.

Next day Andrey Yefimitch was buried. Mihail Averyanitch and Daryushka were the only people at the funeral.

The Grasshopper

All Olga Ivanovna's friends and acquaintances were at her wedding.

"Look at him; isn't it true that there is something in him?" she said to her friends, with a nod towards her husband, as though she wanted to explain why she was marrying a simple, very ordinary, and in no way remarkable man.

Her husband, Osip Stepanitch Dymov, was a doctor, and only of the rank of titular councilor. He was on the staff of two hospitals: in one a ward-surgeon and in the other a dissecting demonstrator. Every day from nine to twelve he saw patients and was busy in his ward, and after twelve o'clock he went by tram to the other hospital, where he dissected. His private practice was a small one, not worth more than five hundred rubles a year. That was all. What more could one say about him? Meanwhile, Olga Ivanovna and her friends and acquaintances were not quite ordinary people. Every one of them was remarkable in some way, and more or less famous; already had made a reputation and was looked upon as a celebrity; or if not yet a celebrity, gave brilliant promise of becoming one. There was an actor from the Dramatic Theatre, who was a great talent of established reputation, as well as an elegant, intelligent, and modest man, and a capital elocutionist, and who taught Olga Ivanovna to recite; there was a singer from the opera, a good-natured, fat man who assured Olga Ivanovna, with a sigh, that she was ruining herself, that if she would take herself in hand and not be lazy she might make a remarkable singer; then there were several artists, and chief among them Ryabovsky, a very handsome, fair young man of five-and-twenty who painted genre pieces, animal studies, and landscapes, was successful at exhibitions, and had sold his last picture for five hundred rubles. He touched up Olga Ivanovna's sketches, and used to say she might do something. Then a violoncellist, whose instrument used to sob, and who openly declared that of all the ladies of his acquaintance the only one who could accompany him was Olga Ivanovna; then there was a literary man, young but already well known, who had written stories, novels, and plays. Who else? Why, Vassily Vassilyitch, a landowner and amateur illustrator and vignettist, with a great feeling for the old Russian style, the old ballad and epic. On paper, on china, and on smoked plates, he produced literally marvels. In the midst of this free artistic company, spoiled by fortune, though refined and modest, who recalled the existence of doctors only in times of illness, and to whom the name Dymov sounded in no way different from Sidorov or Tarasov—in the midst of this company Dymov seemed strange, not wanted, and small, though he was tall and broad-shouldered. He looked as though he had somebody else's coat, and his beard was like a shopman's. Though if he had been a writer or an artist, they would have said that his beard reminded them of Zola.

An artist said to Olga Ivanovna that with her flaxen hair and in her wedding dress she was very much like a graceful cherry tree when it is covered all over with delicate white blossoms in spring.

"Oh, let me tell you," said Olga Ivanovna, taking his arm, "how it was it all came to pass so suddenly. Listen, listen! . . . I must tell you that my father was on the same staff at the hospital as Dymov. When my poor father was taken ill, Dymov watched for days and nights together at his bedside. Such self-sacrifice, such genuine sympathy! I sat up with my father, and did not sleep for nights, either. And all at once—the princess had won the hero's heart—my Dymov fell head over ears in love. Really, fate is so strange at times! Well, after my father's death he came to see me sometimes, met me in the street, and one fine evening, all at once he made me an offer . . . like snow upon my head. . . . I lay awake all night, crying and fell hellishly in love myself. And here, as you see, I am his wife. There really is something strong, powerful, bearlike about him, isn't there? Now his face is turned three-quarters towards us in a bad light, but when he turns round look at his forehead. Ryabovsky, what do you say to that forehead? Dymov, we are talking about you!" she called to her husband. "Come here; hold out your honest hand to Ryabovsky. . . . That's right, be friends."

Dymov, with a naïve and good-natured smile, held out his hand to Ryabovsky, and said:

"Very glad to meet you. There was a Ryabovsky in my year at the medical school. Was he a relation of yours?"

II

Olga Ivanovna was twenty-two, Dymov was thirty-one. They got on splendidly together when they were married. Olga Ivanovna hung all her drawing-room walls with her own and other people's sketches, in frames and without frames, and near the piano and furniture arranged picturesque corners with Japanese parasols, easels, daggers, busts, photographs, and rags of many colors. . . . In the dining room she papered the walls with peasant woodcuts, hung up bark shoes and sickles, stood in a corner a scythe and rake, and so achieved a dining room in the Russian style. In her bedroom she draped the ceiling and the walls with dark cloths to make it like a cavern, hung a Venetian lantern over the beds, and at the door set a figure with a halberd. And everyone thought that the young people had a very charming little home.

When she got up at eleven o'clock every morning, Olga Ivanovna played the piano or, if it were sunny, painted something in oils. Then between twelve and one she drove to her dressmaker's. As Dymov and she had very little money, only just enough, she and her dressmaker were often put to clever shifts to enable her to appear constantly in new dresses and make a sensation with them. Very often out of an old dyed dress, out of bits of tulle, lace, plush, and silk, costing nothing, perfect marvels were created, something bewitching—not a dress, but a dream. From the dressmaker's Olga Ivanovna usually drove to some actress of her acquaintance to hear the latest theatrical gossip, and incidentally to try and get hold of tickets for the first night of some new play or for a benefit performance. From the actress's she had to go to some artist's studio or to some exhibition or to see some celebrity—either to pay a visit or to give an invitation or simply to have a chat. And everywhere she met with a gay and friendly welcome, and was assured that she was good, that she was sweet, that she was rare. . . . Those whom she called great and famous received her as one of themselves, as an equal, and predicted with one voice that, with her talents, her taste, and her intelligence, she would do great things if she concentrated herself. She sang, she played the piano, she painted in oils, she carved, she took part in amateur performances; and all this not just anyhow, but all with talent, whether she made lanterns for an illumination or dressed up or tied somebody's cravat—everything she did was exceptionally graceful, artistic, and charming. But her talents showed themselves in nothing so clearly as in her faculty for quickly becoming acquainted and on intimate terms with celebrated people. No sooner did any one become ever so little celebrated, and set people talking about him, than she made his acquaintance, got on friendly terms the same day, and invited him to her house. Every new acquaintance she made was a veritable fete for her. She adored celebrated people, was proud of them, dreamed of them every night. She craved for them, and never could satisfy her craving. The old ones departed and were forgotten, new ones came to replace them, but to these, too, she soon grew accustomed or was disappointed in them, and began eagerly seeking for fresh great men, finding them and seeking for them again. What for?

Between four and five she dined at home with her husband. His simplicity, good sense, and kind-heartedness touched her and moved her up to enthusiasm. She was constantly jumping up, impulsively hugging his head and showering kisses on it.

"You are a clever, generous man, Dymov," she used to say, "but you have one very serious defect. You take absolutely no interest in art. You don't believe in music or painting."

"I don't understand them," he would say mildly. "I have spent all my life in working at natural science and medicine, and I have never had time to take an interest in the arts."

"But, you know, that's awful, Dymov!"

"Why so? Your friends don't know anything of science or medicine, but you don't reproach them with it. Everyone has his own line. I don't understand landscapes and operas, but the way I look at it is that if one set of sensible people devote their whole lives to them, and other sensible people pay immense sums for them, they must be of use. I don't understand them, but not understanding does not imply disbelieving in them."

"Let me shake your honest hand!"

After dinner Olga Ivanovna would drive off to see her friends, then to a theatre or to a concert, and she returned home after midnight. So it was every day.

On Wednesdays she had "At Homes." The hostess and her guests did not play cards and did not dance, but entertained themselves with various arts. An actor from the Dramatic Theatre recited, a singer sang, artists sketched in the albums of which Olga Ivanovna had a great number, the violoncellist played, and the hostess herself sketched, carved, sang, and played accompaniments. In the intervals between the recitations, music, and singing, they talked and argued about literature, the theatre and painting. There were no ladies, for Olga Ivanovna considered all ladies wearisome and vulgar except actresses and her dressmaker. Not one of these entertainments passed without the hostess starting at every ring at the bell, and saying, with a triumphant expression, "It is he," meaning by "he," of course, some new celebrity. Dymov was not in the drawing room, and no one remembered his existence. But exactly at half-past eleven the door leading into the dining-room opened, and Dymov would appear with his good-natured, gentle smile and say, rubbing his hands:

"Come to supper, gentlemen."

They all went into the dining-room, and every time found on the table exactly the same things: a dish of oysters, a piece of ham or veal, sardines, cheese, caviar mushrooms, vodka, and two decanters of wine.

"My dear *maitre d' hotel!*" Olga Ivanovna would say, clasping her hands with enthusiasm, "you are simply fascinating! My friends, look at his forehead! Dymov, turn your profile. Look! He has the face of a Bengal tiger and an expression as kind and sweet as a gazelle. Ah, the darling!"

The visitors ate, and, looking at Dymov, thought, "He really is a nice fellow"; but they soon forgot about him, and went on talking about the theatre, music, and painting.

The young people were happy, and their life flowed on without a hitch.

The third week of their honeymoon was spent, however, not quite happily—sadly, indeed. Dymov caught erysipelas in the hospital, was in bed for six days, and had to have his beautiful black hair cropped. Olga Ivanovna sat beside him and wept bitterly, but when he was better she put a white handkerchief on his shaven head and began to paint him as a Bedouin. And they were both in good spirits. Three days after he had begun to go back to the hospital he had another mischance.

"I have no luck, little mother," he said one day at dinner. "I had four dissections to do today, and I cut two of my fingers at one. And I did not notice it till I got home."

Olga Ivanovna was alarmed. He smiled, and told her that it did not matter, and that he often cut his hands when he was dissecting.

"I get absorbed, little mother, and grow careless."

Olga Ivanovna dreaded symptoms of blood poisoning, and prayed about it every night, but all went well. And again life flowed on peaceful and happy, free from grief and anxiety.

The present was happy, and to follow it spring was at hand, already smiling in the distance, and promising a thousand delights. There would be no end to their happiness. In April, May and June a summer villa a good distance out of town; walks, sketching, fishing, nightingales; and then from July right on to autumn an artist's tour on the Volga, and in this tour Olga Ivanovna would take part as an indispensable member of the society. She had already had made for her two traveling dresses of linen, had bought paints, brushes, canvases, and a new palette for the journey. Almost every day Ryabovsky visited her to see what progress she was making in her painting; when she showed him her painting, he used to thrust his hands deep into his pockets, compress his lips, sniff, and say:

"Ye—es . . . That cloud of yours is screaming: it's not in the evening light. The foreground is somehow chewed up, and there is something, you know, not the thing. . . . And your cottage is weighed down and whines pitifully. That corner ought to have been taken more in shadow, but on the whole is not bad; I like it."

And the more incomprehensibly he talked, the more readily Olga Ivanovna understood him.

III

After dinner on the second day of Trinity week, Dymov bought some sweets and some savories and went down to the villa to see his wife. He had not seen her for a fortnight, and missed her terribly. As he sat in the train and afterwards as he looked for his villa in a big wood, he felt all the while hungry and weary, and dreamed of how he would have supper in freedom with his wife, then tumble into bed and to sleep. And he was delighted as he looked at his parcel, in which there was caviar, cheese, and white salmon.

The sun was setting by the time he found his villa and recognized it. The old servant told him that her mistress was not at home, but that most likely she would soon be in. The villa, very uninviting in appearance, with low ceilings papered with writing paper and with uneven floors full of crevices consisted only of three rooms. In one there was a bed, in the second there were canvases, brushes, greasy papers, and men's overcoats and hats lying about on the chairs and in the windows, while in the third Dymov found three unknown men; two were dark-haired and had beards, the other was clean-shaven and fat, apparently an actor. There was a samovar boiling on the table.

"What do you want?" asked the actor in a bass voice, looking at Dymov ungraciously. "Do you want Olga Ivanovna? Wait a minute; she will be here directly."

Dymov sat down and waited. One of the dark-haired men, looking sleepily and listlessly at him, poured himself out a glass of tea, and asked:

"Perhaps you would like some tea?"

Dymov was both hungry and thirsty, but he refused tea for fear of spoiling his supper. Soon he heard footsteps and a familiar laugh; a door slammed, and Olga Ivanovna ran into the room, wearing a wide-brimmed hat and carrying a box in her hand; she was followed by Ryabovsky, rosy and good-humored, carrying a big umbrella and a camp-stool.

"Dymov!" cried Olga Ivanovna, and she flushed crimson with pleasure. "Dymov!" she repeated, laying her head and both arms on his bosom. "Is that you? Why haven't you come for so long? Why? Why?"

"When could I, little mother? I am always busy, and whenever I am free it always happens somehow that the train does not fit."

"But how glad I am to see you! I have been dreaming about you the whole night, the whole night, and I was afraid you must be ill. Ah! If you only knew how sweet you are! You have come in the nick of time! You will be my salvation! You are the only person who can save me! There is to be a most original wedding here tomorrow," she went on, laughing, and tying her husband's cravat. "A young telegraph clerk at the station, called Tchikeldyeev, is going to be married. He is a handsome young man and—well, not stupid, and you know there is something strong, bearlike in his face . . . you might paint him as a young Norman. We summer visitors take a great interest in him, and have promised to be at his wedding. . . . He is a lonely, timid man, not well off, and of course it would be a shame not to be sympathetic to him. Fancy! The wedding will be after the service; then we shall all walk from the church to the bride's lodgings . . . you see the wood, the birds singing, patches of sunlight on the grass, and all of us spots of different colors against the bright green background—very original, in the style of the French impressionists. But, Dymov, what am I to go to the church in?" said Olga Ivanovna, and she looked as though she were going to cry. "I have nothing here, literally nothing! No dress, no flowers, no gloves . . . you must save me. Since you have come, fate itself bids you save me. Take the keys, my precious, go home and get my pink dress from the wardrobe. You remember it; it hangs in front. . . . Then, in the storeroom, on the floor, on the right side, you will see two cardboard boxes. When you open the top one you will see tulle, heaps of tulle and rags of all sorts, and under them flowers. Take out all the flowers carefully, try not to crush them, darling; I will choose among them later. . . . And buy me some gloves."

"Very well," said Dymov; "I will go tomorrow and send them to you."

"Tomorrow?" asked Olga Ivanovna, and she looked at him surprised. "You won't have time tomorrow. The first train goes tomorrow at nine, and the wedding's at eleven. No, darling, it must be today; it absolutely must be today. If you won't be able to come tomorrow, send them by a messenger. Come, you must run along. . . . The passenger train will be in directly; don't miss it, darling."

"Very well."

"Oh, how sorry I am to let you go!" said Olga Ivanovna, and tears came into her eyes. "And why did I promise that telegraph clerk, like a silly?"

Dymov hurriedly drank a glass of tea, took a cracknel, and, smiling gently, went to the station. And the caviar, the cheese, and the white salmon were eaten by the two dark gentlemen and the fat actor.

IV

On a still moonlight night in July, Olga Ivanovna was standing on the deck of a Volga steamer and looking alternately at the water and at the picturesque banks. Beside her was standing Ryabovsky, telling her the black shadows on the water were not shadows, but a dream, that it would be sweet to sink into forgetfulness, to die, to become a memory in the sight of that enchanted water with the fantastic glimmer, in sight of the fathomless sky and the mournful, dreamy shores that told of the vanity of our life and of the existence of something higher, blessed, and eternal. The past was vulgar and uninteresting, the future was trivial, and that marvelous night, unique in a lifetime, would soon be over, would blend with eternity; then, why live?

And Olga Ivanovna listened alternately to Ryabovsky's voice and the silence of the night, and thought of her being immortal and never dying. The turquoise color of the water such as she had never seen before, the sky, the river-banks, the black shadows, and the unaccountable joy that flooded her soul, all told her that she would make a great artist, and that somewhere in the distance, in the infinite space beyond the moonlight, success, glory, the love of the people, lay awaiting her. . . . When she gazed steadily without blinking into the distance, she seemed to see crowds of people, lights, triumphant strains of music, cries of enthusiasm, she herself in a white dress, and flowers showered upon her from all sides. She thought, too, that beside her, leaning with his elbow on the rail of the steamer, there was standing a real great man, a genius, one of God's elect. . . . All that he had created up to the present was fine, new, and extraordinary, but what he would create in time, when with maturity his rare talent reached its full development, would be astounding, immeasurably sublime; and that could be seen by his face, by his manner of expressing himself and his attitude to nature. He talked of shadows, of the tones of evening, of the moonlight, in a special way, in a language of his own, so that one could not help feeling the fascination of his power over nature. He was very handsome, original, and his life, free, independent, aloof from all common cares, was like the life of a bird.

"It's growing cooler," said Olga Ivanovna, and she gave a shudder.

Ryabovsky wrapped her in his cloak, and said mournfully:

"I feel that I am in your power; I am a slave. Why are you so enchanting today?"

He kept staring intently at her, and his eyes were terrible. And she was afraid to look at him.

"I love you madly," he whispered, breathing on her cheek. "Say one word to me and I will not go on living; I will give up art. . . ." he muttered in violent emotion. "Love me, love . . ."

"Don't talk like that," said Olga Ivanovna, covering her eyes. "It's dreadful! How about Dymov?"

"What of Dymov? Why Dymov? What have I to do with Dymov? The Volga, the moon, beauty, my love, ecstasy, and there is no such thing as Dymov. . . . Ah! I don't know . . . I don't care about the past; give me one moment, one instant!"

Olga Ivanovna's heart began to throb. She tried to think about her husband, but all her past, with her wedding, with Dymov, and with her "At Homes," seemed to her petty, trivial, dingy, unnecessary, and far, far away. . . . Yes, really, what of Dymov? Why Dymov? What had she to do with Dymov? Had he any existence in nature, or was he only a dream?

"For him, a simple and ordinary man the happiness he has had already is enough," she thought, covering her face with her hands. "Let them condemn me, let them curse me, but in spite of them all I will go to my ruin; I will go to my ruin! . . . One must experience everything in life. My God! How terrible and how glorious!"

"Well? Well?" muttered the artist, embracing her, and greedily kissing the hands with which she feebly tried to thrust him from her. "You love me? Yes? Yes? Oh, what a night! marvelous night!"

"Yes, what a night!" she whispered, looking into his eyes, which were bright with tears.

Then she looked round quickly, put her arms round him, and kissed him on the lips.

"We are nearing Kineshmo!" said someone on the other side of the deck.

They heard heavy footsteps; it was a waiter from the refreshment bar.

"Waiter," said Olga Ivanovna, laughing and crying with happiness, "Bring us some wine."

The artist, pale with emotion, sat on the seat, looking at Olga Ivanovna with adoring, grateful eyes; then he closed his eyes, and said, smiling languidly:

"I am tired."

And he leaned his head against the rail.

V

On the second of September the day was warm and still, but overcast. In the early morning a light mist had hung over the Volga, and after nine o'clock it had begun to spout with rain. And there seemed no hope of the sky clearing. Over their morning tea Ryabovsky told Olga Ivanovna that painting was the most ungrateful and boring art, that he was not an artist, that none but fools thought that he had any talent, and all at once, for no rhyme or reason, he snatched up a knife and with it scraped over his very best sketch. After his tea he sat plunged in gloom at the window and gazed at the Volga. And now the Volga was dingy, all of one even color without a gleam of light, cold-looking. Everything, everything recalled the approach of dreary, gloomy autumn. And it seemed as though nature had removed now from the Volga the sumptuous green covers from the banks, the brilliant reflections of the sunbeams, the transparent blue distance, and all its smart gala array, and had packed it away in boxes till the coming spring, and the crows were flying above the Volga and crying tauntingly, "Bare, bare!"

Ryabovsky heard their cawing, and thought he had already gone off and lost his talent, that everything in this world was relative, conditional, and stupid, and that he ought not to have taken up with this woman. . . . In short, he was out of humor and depressed.

Olga Ivanovna sat behind the screen on the bed, and, passing her fingers through her lovely flaxen hair, pictured herself first in the drawing-room, then in the bedroom, then in her husband's study; her imagination carried her to the theatre, to the dressmaker, to her distinguished friends. Were they getting something up now? Did they think of her? The season had begun by now, and it would be time to think about her "At Homes." And Dymov? Dear Dymov! with what gentleness and childlike pathos he kept begging her in his letters to make haste and come home! Every month he sent her seventy-five rubles, and when she wrote him that she had lent the artists a hundred rubles, he sent that hundred too. What a kind, generous-hearted man! The traveling wearied Olga Ivanovna; she was bored; and she longed to get away from the peasants, from the damp smell of the river, and to cast off the feeling of physical uncleanliness of which she was conscious all the time, living in the peasants' huts and wandering from village to village. If Ryabovsky had not given his word to the artists that he would stay with them till the twentieth of September they might have gone away that very day. And how nice that would have been!

"My God!" moaned Ryabovsky. "Will the sun ever come out? I can't go on with a sunny landscape without the sun. . . ."

"But you have a sketch with a cloudy sky," said Olga Ivanovna, coming from behind the screen. "Do you remember, in the right foreground forest trees, on the left a herd of cows and geese? You might finish it now."

"Aie!" the artist scowled. "Finish it! Can you imagine I am such a fool that I don't know what I want to do?"

"How you have changed to me!" sighed Olga Ivanovna.

"Well, a good thing too!"

Olga Ivanovna's face quivered; she moved away to the stove and began to cry.

"Well, that's the last straw—crying! Give over! I have a thousand reasons for tears, but I am not crying."

"A thousand reasons!" cried Olga Ivanovna. "The chief one is that you are weary of me. Yes!" she said, and broke into sobs. "If one is to tell the truth, you are ashamed of our love. You keep trying to prevent the artists from noticing it though it is impossible to conceal it, and they have known all about if for ever so long."

"Olga, one thing I beg you," said the artist in an imploring voice, laying his hand on his heart—"one thing; don't worry me! I want nothing else from you!"

"But swear that you love me still!"

"This is agony!" the artist hissed through his teeth, and he jumped up. "It will end by my throwing myself in the Volga or going out of my mind! Let me alone!"

"Come, kill me, kill me!" cried Olga Ivanovna. "Kill me!"

She sobbed again, and went behind the screen. There was a swish of rain on the straw thatch of the hut. Ryabovsky clutched his head and strode as though bent on proving something to somebody, put on his cap, slung his gun over his shoulder, and went out of the hut.

After he had gone, Olga Ivanovna lay a long time on the bed, crying. At first she thought it would be a good thing to poison herself, so that when Ryabovsky came back he would find her dead; then her imagination carried her to her drawing-room, to her husband's study, and she imagined herself sitting motionless beside Dymov and enjoying the physical peace and cleanliness, and in the evening sitting in the theatre, listening to Mazini. And a yearning for civilization, for the noise and bustle of the town, for celebrated people sent a pang to her heart. A peasant woman came into the hut and began in a leisurely way lighting the stove to get the dinner. There was a smell of charcoal fumes, and the air was filled with bluish smoke. The artists came in, in muddy high boots and with faces wet with rain, examined their sketches, and comforted themselves by saying that the Volga had its charms even in bad weather. On the wall the cheap clock went "tic-tic-tic." The flies, feeling chilled, crowded round the icon in the corner, buzzing, and one could hear the cockroaches scurrying about among the thick portfolios under the seats. . . .

Ryabovsky came home as the sun was setting. He flung his cap on the table, and, without removing his muddy boots, sank pale and exhausted on the bench and closed his eyes.

"I am tired," he said, and twitched his eyebrows, trying to raise his eyelids.

To be nice to him and to show she was not cross, Olga Ivanovna went up to him, gave him a silent kiss, and passed the comb through his fair hair. She meant to comb it for him.

"What's that?" he said, starting as though something cold had touched him, and he opened his eyes. "What is it? Please let me alone."

He thrust her off, and moved away. And it seemed to her that there was a look of aversion and annoyance on his face.

At that time the peasant woman cautiously carried him, in both hands, a plate of cabbage-soup. And Olga Ivanovna saw how she wetted her fat fingers in it. And the dirty peasant woman, standing with her body thrust forward, and the cabbage-soup, which Ryabovsky began eating greedily, and the hut, and their whole way of life, which she at first had so loved for its simplicity and artistic disorder, seemed horrible to her now. She suddenly felt insulted, and said coldly:

"We must part for a time, or else from boredom we shall quarrel in earnest. I am sick of this; I am going today."

"Going how? Astride on a broomstick?"

"Today is Thursday, so the steamer will be here at half-past nine."

"Eh? Yes, yes. . . . Well, go, then. . . ." Ryabovsky said softly, wiping his mouth with a towel instead of a dinner napkin. "You are dull and have nothing to do here, and one would have to be a great egoist to try and keep you. Go home, and we shall meet again after the twentieth."

Olga Ivanovna packed in good spirits. Her cheeks positively glowed with pleasure. Could it really be true, she asked herself, that she would soon be writing in her drawing room and sleeping in her bedroom, and dining with a cloth on the table? A weight was lifted from her heart, and she no longer felt angry with the artist.

"My paints and brushes I will leave with you, Ryabovsky," she said. "You can bring what's left. . . . Mind, now, don't be lazy here when I am gone; don't mope, but work. You are such a splendid fellow, Ryabovsky!"

At ten o'clock Ryabovsky gave her a farewell kiss, in order, as she thought, to avoid kissing her on the steamer before the artists, and went with her to the landing stage. The steamer soon came up and carried her away.

She arrived home two and a half days later. Breathless with excitement, she went, without taking off her hat or waterproof, into the drawing room and thence into the dining room. Dymov, with his waistcoat unbuttoned and no coat, was sitting at the table sharpening a knife on a fork; before him lay a grouse on a plate. As Olga Ivanovna went into the flat she was convinced that it was essential to hide everything from her husband, and that she would have the strength and skill to do so; but now, when she saw his broad, mild, happy smile, and shining, joyful eyes, she felt that to deceive this man was as vile, as revolting, and as impossible and out of her power as to bear false witness, to steal, or to kill, and in a flash she resolved to tell him all that had happened. Letting him kiss and embrace her, she sank down on her knees before him and hid her face.

"What is it, what is it, little mother?" he asked tenderly. "Were you homesick?"

She raised her face, red with shame, and gazed at him with a guilty and imploring look, but fear and shame prevented her from telling him the truth.

"Nothing," she said; "it's just nothing. . . ."

"Let us sit down," he said, raising her and seating her at the table. "That's right, eat the grouse. You are starving, poor darling."

She eagerly breathed in the atmosphere of home and ate the grouse, while he watched her with tenderness and laughed with delight.

.

VI

Apparently by the middle of winter Dymov began to suspect that he was being deceived. As though his conscience was not clear, he could not look his wife straight in the face, did not smile with delight when he met her, and to avoid being left alone with her, he often brought in to dinner his colleague, Korostelev, a little close-cropped man with a wrinkled face, who kept buttoning and unbuttoning his reefer jacket with embarrassment when he talked with Olga Ivanovna, and then with his right hand nipped his left moustache. At dinner the two doctors talked about the fact that a displacement of the diaphragm was sometimes accompanied by irregularities of the heart, or that a great number of neurotic complaints were met with of late or that Dymov had the day before found a cancer of the lower abdomen while dissecting a corpse with the diagnosis of pernicious anemia. And it seemed as though they were talking of medicine to give Olga

Ivanovna a chance of being silent—that is, of not lying. After dinner Korostelev sat down to the piano, while Dymov sighed and said to him:

"Ech, brother—well, well! Play something melancholy."

Hunching up his shoulders and stretching his fingers wide apart, Korostelev played some chords and began singing in a tenor voice, "Show me the abode where the Russian peasant would not groan," while Dymov sighed once more, propped his head on his fist, and sank into thought.

Olga Ivanovna had been extremely imprudent in her conduct of late. Every morning she woke up in a very bad humor and with the thought that she no longer cared for Ryabovsky, and that, thank God, it was all over now. But as she drank her coffee she reflected that Ryabovsky had robbed her of her husband, and that now she was left with neither her husband nor Ryabovsky; then she remembered talks she had heard among her acquaintances of a picture Ryabovsky was preparing for the exhibition, something striking, a mixture of genre and landscape, in the style of Polyenov, about which everyone who had been into his studio went into raptures; and this, of course, she mused, he had created under her influence, and altogether, thanks to her influence, he had greatly changed for the better. Her influence was so beneficent and essential that if she were to leave him he might perhaps go to ruin. And she remembered, too, that the last time he had come to see her in a great-coat with flecks on it and a new tie, he had asked her languidly:

"Am I beautiful?"

And with his elegance, his long curls, and his blue eyes, he really was very beautiful (or perhaps it only seemed so), and he had been affectionate to her.

Considering and remembering many things Olga Ivanovna dressed and in great agitation drove to Ryabovsky's studio. She found him in high spirits, and enchanted with his really magnificent picture. He was dancing about and playing the fool and answering serious questions with jokes. Olga Ivanovna was jealous of the picture and hated it, but from politeness she stood before the picture for five minutes in silence, and, heaving a sigh, as though before a holy shrine, said softly:

"Yes, you have never painted anything like it before. Do you know it is positively awe-inspiring?"

And then she began beseeching him to love her and not to cast her off, to have pity on her in her misery and her wretchedness. She shed tears, kissed his hands, insisted on his swearing that he love her, told him that without her good influence he would go astray and be ruined. And, when she had spoilt his good humor, feeling herself humiliated, she would drive off to her dressmaker or to an actress of her acquaintance to try and get theatre tickets.

If she did not find him at his studio she left a letter in which she swore that if he did not come to see her that day she would poison herself. He was scared, came to see her, and stayed to dinner. Regardless of her husband's presence, he would say rude things to her, and she would answer him in the same way. Both felt they were a burden to each other, that they were tyrants and enemies, and were wrathful, and in their wrath did not notice that their behavior was unseemly, and that even Korostelev, with his close-cropped head, saw it all. After dinner Ryabovsky made haste to say good-by and get away.

"Where are you off to?" Olga Ivanovna would ask him in the hall, looking at him with hatred.

Scowling and screwing up his eyes, he mentioned some lady of their acquaintance, and it was evident that he was laughing at her jealousy and wanted to annoy her. She went to her bedroom and lay down on her bed; from jealousy, anger, a sense of humiliation and shame, she bit the pillow and began sobbing aloud. Dymov left Korostelev in the drawing room, went into the bedroom, and with a desperate and embarrassed face said softly:

"Don't cry so loud, little mother; there's no need. You must be quiet about it. You must not let people see. . . . You know what is done is done, and can't be mended."

Not knowing how to ease the burden of her jealousy, which actually set her temples throbbing with pain, and thinking still that things might be set right, she would wash, powder her tear-stained face, and fly off to the lady mentioned.

Not finding Ryabovsky with her, she would drive off to a second, then to a third. At first she was ashamed to go about like this, but afterwards she got used to it, and it would happen that in one evening she would make the round of all her female acquaintances in search of Ryabovsky, and they all understood it.

One day she said to Ryabovsky of her husband:

"That man crushes me with his magnanimity."

This phrase pleased her so much that when she met with artists who knew of her affair with Ryabovsky she said every time of her husband, with a vigorous movement of her arm:

"That man crushes me with his magnanimity."

Their manner of life was the same as it had been the year before. On Wednesdays they were "At Home"; an actor recited, the artists sketched. The violoncellist played, a singer sang, and invariably at half-past eleven the door leading to the dining-room opened and Dymov, smiling, said:

"Come to supper, gentlemen."

As before, Olga Ivanovna hunted celebrities, found them, was not satisfied, and went in pursuit of fresh ones. As before, she came back late every night; but now Dymov was not, as last year, asleep, but sitting in his study at work of some sort. He went to bed at three o'clock and got up at eight.

One evening when she was getting ready to go to the theatre and standing before the pier glass, Dymov came into her bedroom, wearing his dress-coat and a white tie. He was smiling gently and looked into his wife's face joyfully, as in old days; his face was radiant.

"I have just been defending my thesis," he said, sitting down and smoothing his knees.

"Defending?" asked Olga Ivanovna.

"Oh oh!" he laughed, and he craned his neck to see his wife's face in the mirror for she was still standing with her back to him, doing up her hair. "Oh, oh," he repeated, "do you know it's very possible they may offer me the Readership in General Pathology? It seems like it."

It was evident from his beaming, blissful face that if Olga Ivanovna had shared with him his joy and triumph he would have forgiven her everything, both the present and the future, and would have forgotten everything, but she did not understand what was meant by a "readership" or by "general pathology"; besides, she was afraid of being late for the theatre and she said nothing.

He sat there another two minutes, and with a guilty smile went away.

VII

It had been a very troubled day.

Dymov had a very bad headache; he had no breakfast, and did not go to the hospital, but spent the whole time lying on his sofa in the study. Olga Ivanovna went as usual at midday to see Ryabovsky, to show him her still-life sketch, and to ask him why he had not been to see her the evening before. The sketch seemed to her worthless, and she had painted it only in order to have an additional reason for going to the artist.

She went in to him without ringing, and as she was taking off her galoshes in the entry she heard a sound as of something running softly in the studio, with a feminine rustle of skirts; and as she hastened to peep in she caught a momentary glimpse of a bit of brown petticoat, which vanished behind a big picture draped, together with the easel, with black calico, to the floor. There could be no doubt that a woman was hiding there. How often Olga Ivanovna herself had taken refuge behind that picture!

Ryabovsky, evidently much embarrassed, held out both hands to her, as though surprised at her arrival and said with a forced smile:

"Aha! Very glad to see you! Anything nice to tell me?"

Olga Ivanovna's eyes filled with tears. She felt ashamed and bitter, and would not for a million rubles have consented to speak in the presence of the outsider, the rival, the deceitful woman who was standing now behind the picture, and probably giggling malignantly.

"I have brought you a sketch," she said timidly in a thin voice, and her lips quivered. "*Nature morte.*"

"Ah—ah! . . . A sketch?"

The artist took the sketch in his hands, and as he examined it walked, as it were mechanically, into the other room.

Olga Ivanovna followed him humbly.

"*Nature morte* . . . first-rate sort," he muttered, falling into rhyme. "Kurort . . . sport . . . port . . ."

From the studio came the sound of hurried footsteps and the rustle of a skirt.

So she had gone. Olga Ivanovna wanted to scream aloud, to hit the artist on the head with something heavy, but she could see nothing through her tears, was crushed by her shame, and felt herself, not Olga Ivanovna, not an artist, but a little insect.

"I am tired. . . ." said the artist languidly, looking at the sketch and tossing his head as though struggling with drowsiness. "It's very nice, of course, but here a sketch today, a sketch last year, another sketch in a month . . . I wonder you are not bored with them. If I were you I should give up painting and work seriously at music or something. You're not an artist, you know, but a musician. But you can't think how tired I am! I'll tell them to bring us some tea, shall I?"

He went out of the room, and Olga Ivanovna heard him give some order to his footman. To avoid farewells and explanations, and above all to avoid bursting into sobs, she ran as fast as she could, before Ryabovsky came back, to the entry, put on her galoshes, and went out into the street; then she breathed easily and felt she was free forever from Ryabovsky and from painting and from the burden of shame which had so crushed her in the studio. It was all over!

She drove to her dressmaker's; then to see Barnay, who had only arrived the day before; from Barnay to a music-shop, and all the time she was thinking how she would write Ryabovsky a cold, cruel letter full of personal dignity, and how in the spring or the summer she would go with Dymov to the Crimea, free herself finally from the past there, and begin a new life.

On getting home late in the evening she sat down in the drawing room, without taking off her things, to begin the letter. Ryabovsky had told her she was not an artist, and to pay him out she wrote to him now that he painted the same thing every year, and said exactly the same thing every day; that he was at a standstill, and that nothing more would come of him than had come already. She wanted to write, too, that he owed a great deal to her good influence, and that if he was going wrong it was only because her influence was paralyzed by various dubious persons like the one who had been hiding behind the picture that day.

"Little mother!" Dymov called from the study, without opening the door. "What is it?"

"Don't come in to me, but only come to the door—that's right. . . . the day before yesterday I must have caught diphtheria at the hospital, and now . . . I am ill. Make haste and send for Korostelev." Olga Ivanovna always called her husband by his surname, as she did all the men of her acquaintance; she disliked his Christian name, Osip, because it reminded her of the Osip in Gogol and the silly pun on his name. But now she cried:

"Osip, it cannot be!"

"Send for him; I feel ill," Dymov said behind the door, and she could hear him go back to the sofa and lie down. "Send!" she heard his voice faintly.

"Good Heavens!" thought Olga Ivanovna, turning chill with horror. "Why, it's dangerous!"

For no reason she took the candle and went into the bedroom, and there, reflecting what she must do, glanced casually at herself in the pier glass. With her pale, frightened face, in a jacket with sleeves high on the shoulders, with yellow ruches on her bosom, and with stripes running in unusual directions on her skirt, she seemed to herself horrible and disgusting. She suddenly felt poignantly sorry for Dymov, for his boundless love for her, for his young life, and even for the desolate little bed in which he had not slept for so long; and she remembered his habitual, gentle, submissive smile. She wept bitterly, and wrote an imploring letter to Korostelev. It was two o'clock in the night.

VIII

When towards eight o'clock in the morning Olga Ivanovna, her head heavy from want of sleep and her hair unbrushed, came out of her bedroom, looking unattractive and with a guilty expression on her face, a gentleman with a black beard, apparently the doctor, passed by her into the entry. There was a smell of drugs. Korostelev was standing near the study door, twisting his left moustache with his right hand.

"Excuse me, I can't let you go in," he said surily to Olga Ivanovna; "it's catching. Besides, it's no use, really; he is delirious, anyway."

"Has he really got diphtheria?" Olga Ivanovna asked in a whisper.

"People who wantonly risk infection ought to be hauled up and punished for it," muttered Korostelev, not answering Olga Ivanovna's question. "Do you know why he caught it? On Tuesday he was sucking up the mucus through a pipette from a boy with diphtheria. And what for? It was stupid. . . . Just from folly. . . ."

"Is it dangerous, very?" asked Olga Ivanovna.

"Yes; they say it is the malignant form. We ought to send for Shrek really."

A little red-haired man with a long nose and a Jewish accent arrived; then a tall, stooping, shaggy individual, who looked like a head deacon; then a stout young man with a red face and spectacles. These were doctors who came to watch by turns beside their colleague. Korostelev did not go home when his turn was over, but remained and wandered about the rooms like an uneasy spirit. The maid kept getting tea for the various doctors, and was constantly running to the chemist, and there was no one to do the rooms. There was a dismal stillness in the flat.

Olga Ivanovna sat in her bedroom and thought that God was punishing her for having deceived her husband. That silent, unrepining, uncomprehended creature, robbed by his mildness of all personality and will, weak from excessive kindness, had been suffering in obscurity somewhere on his sofa, and had not complained. And if he were to complain even in delirium, the doctors watching by his bedside would learn that diphtheria was not the only cause of his sufferings. They would ask Korostelev. He knew all about it, and it was not for nothing that he looked at his friend's wife with eyes that seemed to say that she was the real chief criminal and diphtheria was only her accomplice. She did not think now of the moonlight evening on the Volga, nor the words of love, nor their poetical life in the peasant's hut. She thought only that from an idle whim, from self-indulgence, she had sullied herself all over from head to foot in something filthy, sticky, which one could never wash off. . . .

"Oh, how fearfully false I've been!" she thought, recalling the troubled passion she had known with Ryabovsky. "Curse it all!"

At four o'clock she dined with Korostelev. He did nothing but scowl and drink red wine, and did not eat a morsel. She ate nothing, either. At one minute she was praying inwardly and vowing to God that if Dymov recovered she would love him again and be a faithful wife to him. Then, forgetting herself for a minute, she would look at Korostelev, and think: "Surely it must be dull to be a humble, obscure person, not remarkable in any way, especially with such a wrinkled face and bad manners!" Then it seemed to her that God would strike her dead that minute for not having once been in her husband's study, for fear of infection. And altogether she had a dull, despondent feeling and a conviction that her life was spoilt, and that there was no setting it right anyhow.

After dinner darkness came on. When Olga Ivanovna went into the drawing-room Korostelev was asleep on the sofa, with a gold-embroidered silk cushion under his head.

"Khee-poo-ah," he snored—"khee-poo-ah."

And the doctors as they came to sit up and went away again did not notice this disorder. The fact that a strange man was asleep and snoring in the drawing-room, and the sketches on the walls and the exquisite decoration of the room, and the fact that the lady of the house was disheveled and untidy—all that aroused not the slightest interest now. One of the doctors chanced to laugh at something, and the laugh had a strange and timid sound that made one's heart ache.

When Olga Ivanovna went into the drawing room next time, Korostelev was not asleep, but sitting up and smoking.

"He has diphtheria of the nasal cavity," he said in a low voice, "and the heart is not working properly now. Things are in a bad way, really."

"But you will send for Shrek?" said Olga Ivanovna.

"He has been already. It was he who noticed that the diphtheria had passed into the nose. What's the use of Shrek! Shrek's no use at all, really. He is Shrek, I am Korostelev, and nothing more."

The time dragged on fearfully slowly. Olga Ivanovna lay down in her clothes on her bed, that had not been made all day, and sank into a doze. She dreamed that the whole flat was filled up from floor to ceiling with a huge piece of iron, and that if they could only get the iron out they would all be light-hearted and happy. Waking, she realized that it was not the iron but Dymov's illness that was weighing on her.

"Nature morte, port..." she thought, sinking into forgetfulness again. "Sport ... Kurort ... and what of Shrek? Shrek ... trek ... wreck. ... And where are my friends now? Do they know that we are in trouble? Lord, save ... spare! Shrek ... trek ..."

And again the iron was there. ... The time dragged on slowly, though the clock on the lower story struck frequently. And bells were continually ringing as the doctors arrived. ... The housemaid came in with an empty glass on a tray, and asked, "Shall I make the bed, madam?" and getting no answer, went away.

The clock below struck the hour. She dreamed of the rain on the Volga; and again some one came into her bedroom, she thought a stranger. Olga Ivanovna jumped up, and recognized Korostelev.

"What time is it?" she asked.

"About three."

"Well, what is it?"

"What, indeed! ... I've come to tell you he is passing. ..."

He gave a sob, sat down on the bed beside her, and wiped away the tears with his sleeve. She could not grasp it at once, but turned cold all over and began slowly crossing herself.

"He is passing," he repeated in a shrill voice, and again he gave a sob. "He is dying because he sacrificed himself. What a loss for science!" he said bitterly. "Compare him with all of us. He was a great man, an extraordinary man! What gifts! What hopes we all had of him!" Korostelev went on, wringing his hands: "Merciful God, he was a man of science; we shall never look on his like again. Osip Dymov, what have you done—aie, aie, my God!"

Korostelev covered his face with both hands in despair, and shook his head.

"And his moral force," he went on, seeming to grow more and more exasperated against some one. "Not a man, but a pure, good, loving soul, and clean as crystal. He served science and died for science. And he worked like an ox night and day—no one spared him—and with his youth and his learning he had to take a private practice and work at translations at night to pay for these . . . vile rags!"

Korostelev looked with hatred at Olga Ivanovna, snatched at the sheet with both hands and angrily tore it, as though it were to blame.

"He did not spare himself, and others did not spare him. Oh, what's the use of talking!"

"Yes, he was a rare man," said a bass voice in the drawing room.

Olga Ivanovna remembered her whole life with him from beginning to the end, with all its details, and suddenly she understood that he really was an extraordinary, rare, and, compared with every one else she knew, a great man. And remembering how her father, now dead, and all the other doctors had behaved to him, she realized that they really had seen in him a future celebrity. The walls, the ceiling, the lamp, and the carpet on the floor, seemed to be winking at her sarcastically, as though they would say, "You were blind! You were blind!" With a wail she flung herself out of the bedroom, dashed by some unknown man in the drawing room, and ran into her husband's study. He was lying motionless on the sofa, covered to the waist with a quilt. His face was fearfully thin and sunken, and was of a grayish-yellow color such as is never seen in the living; only from the forehead, from the black eyebrows and from the familiar smile, could he be recognized as Dymov. Olga Ivanovna hurriedly felt his chest, his forehead, and his hands. The chest was still warm, but the forehead and hands were unpleasantly cold, and the half open eyes looked, not at Olga Ivanovna, but at the quilt.

"Dymov!" she called aloud, "Dymov!" She wanted to explain to him that it had been a mistake, that all was not lost, that life might still be beautiful and happy, that he was an extraordinary, rare, great man, and that she would all her life worship him and bow down in homage and holy awe before him. . . .

"Dymov!" she called him, patting him on the shoulder, unable to believe that he would never wake again. "Dymov! Dymov!"

In the drawing room Korostelev was saying to the housemaid:

"Why keep asking? Go to the church beadle and enquire where they live. They'll wash the body and lay it out, and do everything that is necessary."

The Head Gardener's Story

A sale of flowers was taking place in Count N.'s greenhouses. The purchasers were few in number—a landowner who was a neighbor of mine, a young timber merchant, and myself. While the workmen were carrying out our magnificent purchases and packing them into the carts, we sat at the entry of the greenhouse and chatted about one thing and another. It is extremely pleasant to sit in a garden on a still April morning, listening to the birds, and watching the flowers brought out into the open air and basking in the sunshine.

The head gardener, Mihail Karlovitch, a venerable old man with a full shaven face, wearing a fur waistcoat and no coat, superintended the packing of the plants himself, but at the same time he listened to our conversation in the hope of hearing something new. He was an intelligent, very good-hearted man, respected by everyone. He was for some reason looked upon by everyone as a German, though he was in reality on his father's side Swedish, on his mother's side Russian, and attended the Orthodox church. He knew Russian, Swedish, and German. He had read a good deal in those languages, and nothing one could do gave him greater pleasure than lending him some new book or talking to him, for instance, about Ibsen.

He had his weakness, but they were innocent ones: he called himself the head gardener, though there were no under-gardeners; the expression of his face was unusually dignified and haughty; he could not endure to be contradicted, and liked to be listened to with respect and attention.

"That young fellow there I can recommend to you as an awful rascal," said my neighbor, pointing to a laborer with a swarthy, gipsy face, who drove by with the water barrel. "Last week he was tried in town for burglary and was acquitted; they pronounced him mentally deranged, and yet look at him, he is the picture of health. Scoundrels are very often acquitted nowadays in Russia on grounds of abnormality and aberration, yet these acquittals, these unmistakable proofs of an indulgent attitude to crime, lead to no good. They demoralize the masses, the sense of justice is blunted in all as they become accustomed to seeing vice unpunished, and you know in our age one may boldly say in the words of Shakespeare that in our evil and corrupt age virtue must ask forgiveness of vice."

"That's very true," the merchant assented. "Owing to these frequent acquittals, murder and arson have become much more common. Ask the peasants."

Mihail Karlovitch turned towards us and said:

"As far as I am concerned, gentlemen, I am always delighted to meet with these verdicts of not guilty. I am not afraid for morality and justice when they say 'Not guilty,' but on the contrary I feel pleased. Even when my conscience tells me the jury has made a mistake in acquitting the criminal, even then I am triumphant. Judge for yourselves, gentlemen; if the judges and the jury have more faith in *man* than in evidence, material proofs, and speeches for the prosecution, is not that faith *in man* in itself higher than any ordinary considerations? Such faith is only attainable by those few who understand and feel Christ."

"A fine thought," I said.

"But it's not a new one. I remember a very long time ago I heard a legend on that subject. A very charming legend," said the gardener, and he smiled. "I was told it by my grandmother, my father's mother, an excellent old lady. She told me it in Swedish, and it does not sound so fine, so classical, in Russian."

But we begged him to tell it and not to be put off by the coarseness of the Russian language. Much gratified, he deliberately lighted his pipe, looked angrily at the laborers and began:

"There settled in a certain little town a solitary, plain, elderly gentleman called Thomson or Wilson—but that does not matter; the surname is not the point. He followed an honorable profession: he was a doctor. He was always morose and unsociable, and only spoke when required by his profession. He never visited anyone, never extended his acquaintance beyond a silent bow, and lived as humbly as a hermit. The fact was, he was a learned man, and in those days learned men were not like other people. They spent their days and nights in contemplation, reading and in healing disease, looked upon everything else as trivial, and had no time to waste a word. The inhabitants of the town understood this, and tried not to worry him with their visits and empty chatter. They were very glad that God had sent them at last a man who could heal diseases, and were proud that such a remarkable man was living in their town. 'He knows everything,' they said about him.

"But that was not enough. They ought to have also said, 'He loves everyone.' In the breast of that learned man there beat a wonderful angelic heart. Though the people of that town were strangers and not his own people, yet he loved them like children, and did not spare himself for them. He was himself ill with consumption, he had a cough, but when he was summoned to the sick he forgot his own illness, he did not spare himself and, gasping for breath, climbed up the hills however high they might be. He disregarded the sultry heat and the cold, despised thirst and hunger. He would accept no money and, strange to say, when one of his patients died, he would follow the coffin with the relations, weeping.

"And soon he became so necessary to the town that the inhabitants wondered how they could have got on before without the man. Their gratitude knew no bounds. Grown-up people and children, good and bad alike, honest men and cheats—all, in fact, respected him and knew his value. In the little town and the entire surrounding neighborhood there was no man who would allow himself to do anything disagreeable to him; indeed, they would never have dreamed of it. When he came out of his lodging, he never fastened the doors or windows, in complete confidence that there was no thief who could bring himself to do him wrong. He often had in the course of his medical duties to walk along the high-roads, through the forests and mountains haunted by numbers of hungry vagrants; but he felt that he was in perfect security.

"One night he was returning from a patient when robbers fell upon him in the forest, but when they recognized him, they took off their hats respectfully and offered him something to eat. When he answered that he was not hungry, they gave him a warm wrap and accompanied him as far as the town, happy that fate had given them the chance in some small way to show their gratitude to the be-nevolent man. Well, to be sure, my grandmother told me that even the horses and the cows and the dogs knew him and expressed their joy when they met him.

"And this man who seemed by his sanctity to have guarded himself from the evil, to whom even brigands and frenzied men wished nothing but good, was one fine morning found murdered. Covered with blood, with his skull broken, he was lying in a ravine, and his pale face wore an expression of amazement. Yes, not horror but amazement was the emotion that had been fixed upon his face when he saw the murderer before him. You can imagine the grief that overwhelmed the inhabitants of the town and the surrounding districts. All were in despair, unable to believe their eyes, wondering who could have killed the man. The judges who conducted the inquiry and examined the doctor's body said: 'Here we have all the signs of a murder, but as there is not a man in the world capable of mur-dering our doctor, obviously it was not a case of murder, and the combination of evidence is due to simple chance. We must suppose that in the darkness he fell into the ravine of himself and was mortally injured.'

"The whole town agreed with this opinion. The doctor was buried, and noth-ing more was said about a violent death. The existence of a man who could have the baseness and wickedness to kill the doctor seemed incredible. There is a limit even to wickedness, isn't there?

"All at once, would you believe it, chance led them to discovering the mur-derer. A vagrant who had been many times convicted, notorious for his vicious life, was seen selling for drink a snuff-box and watch that had belonged to the doctor. When he was questioned he was confused, and answered with an obvious lie. A search was made, and in his bed was found a shirt with stains of blood on the sleeves, and a doctor's lancet set in gold. What more evidence was wanted? They put the criminal in prison. The inhabitants were indignant, and at the same time said:

"'It's incredible! It can't be so! Take care that a mistake is not made; it does happen, you know, that evidence tells a false tale.'

"At his trial the murderer obstinately denied his guilt. Everything was against him, and to be convinced of his guilt was as easy as to believe that this earth is black; but the judges seem to have gone mad: they weighed every proof ten times, looked distrustfully at the witnesses, flushed crimson and sipped water. . . . The trial began early in the morning and was only finished in the evening.

"'Accused!' the chief judge said, addressing the murderer, 'the court has found you guilty of murdering Dr. So-and-so, and has sentenced you to . . .'"

"The chief judge meant to say 'to the death penalty,' but he dropped from his hands the paper on which the sentence was written, wiped the cold sweat from his face, and cried out:

"'No! May God punish me if I judge wrongly, but I swear he is not guilty. I cannot admit the thought that there exists a man who would dare to murder our friend the doctor! A man could not sink so low!'

"'There cannot be such a man!' the other judges assented.

"'No,' the crowd cried. 'Let him go!'

"The murderer was set free to go where he chose, and not one soul blamed the court for an unjust verdict. And my grandmother used to say that for such faith in humanity God forgave the sins of all the inhabitants of that town. He rejoices when people believe that man is His image and semblance, and grieves if, forgetful of human dignity, they judge worse of men than of dogs. The sentence of acquittal may bring harm to the inhabitants of the town, but on the other hand, think of the beneficial influence upon them of that faith in man—a faith which does not remain dead, you know; it raises up generous feelings in us, and always impels us to love and respect every man. Every man! And that is important."

Mikhail Karlovitch had finished. My neighbor would have urged some objection, but the head gardener made a gesture that signified that he did not like objections; then he walked away to the carts, and, with an expression of dignity, went on looking after the packing.

Ionitch

When visitors to the provincial town S——complained of the dreariness and monotony of life, the inhabitants of the town, as though defending themselves, declared that it was very nice in S——, that there was a library, a theatre, a club; that they had balls; and finally, that there were clever, agreeable, and interesting families with whom one could make acquaintance. And they used to point to the family of the Turkins as the most highly cultivated and talented.

This family lived in their own house in the principal street, near the Governor's. Ivan Petrovitch Turkin himself—a stout, handsome, dark man with whiskers—used to get up amateur performances for benevolent objects, and used to take the part of an elderly general and cough very amusingly. He knew a number of anecdotes, charades, proverbs, and was fond of being humorous and witty, and he always wore an expression from which it was impossible to tell whether he were joking or in earnest. His wife, Vera Iosifovna—a thin, nice-looking lady who wore a pince-nez—used to write novels and stories, and was very fond of reading them aloud to her visitors. The daughter, Ekaterina Ivanovna, a young girl, used to play on the piano. In short, every member of the family had a special talent. The Turkins welcomed visitors, and good-humoredly displayed their talents with genuine simplicity. The stone house was roomy and cool in summer; half of the windows looked into a shady old garden, where nightingales used to sing in the spring. When there were visitors in the house, there was a clatter of knives in the kitchen and a smell of fried onions in the yard—and that was always a sure sign of a plentiful and savory supper to follow.

And as soon as Dmitri Ionitch Startsev was appointed the district doctor, and took up his abode at Dyalizh, six miles from S——, he, too, was told that as a cultivated man it was essential for him to make the acquaintance of the Turkins. In the winter he was introduced to Ivan Petrovitch in the street; they talked about the weather, about the theatre, about the cholera; an invitation followed. On a holiday in the spring—it was Ascension Day—after seeing his patients, Startsev set off for town in search of a little recreation and to make some purchases. He walked in a leisurely way (he had not yet set up his carriage), humming all the time:

"'Before I'd drunk the tears from life's goblet ... '"

In town he dined, went for a walk in the gardens, then Ivan Petrovitch's invitation came into his mind, as it were of itself, and he decided to call on the Turkins and see what sort of people they were.

"How do you do, if you please?" said Ivan Petrovitch, meeting him on the steps. "Delighted, delighted to see such agreeable visitor. Come along; I will introduce you to my better half. I tell him, Verotchka," he went on, as he presented the doctor to his wife—"I tell him that he has no human right to sit at home in a hospital; he ought to devote his leisure to society. Oughtn't he, darling?"

"Sit here," said Vera Iosifovna, making her visitor sit down beside her. "You can dance attendance on me. My husband is jealous—he is an Othello; but we will try and behave so well that he will notice nothing."

"Ah, you spoilt chicken!" Ivan Petrovitch muttered tenderly, and he kissed her on the forehead. "You have come just in the nick of time," he said addressing the doctor again. "My better half has written a 'hugeous' novel, and she is going to read it aloud today."

"Petit Jean," said Vera Iosifovna to her husband, "dites que l'on nous donne du thé."

Startsev was introduced to Ekaterina Ivanovna, a girl of eighteen, very much like her mother, thin and pretty. Her expression was still childish and her figure was soft and slim; and her developed girlish bosom, healthy and beautiful, was suggestive of spring, real spring.

Then they drank tea with jam, honey, and sweetmeats, and with very nice cakes, which melted in the mouth. As the evening came on, other visitors gradually arrived, and Ivan Petrovitch fixed his laughing eyes on each of them and said:

"How do you do, if you please?"

Then they all sat down in the drawing-room with very serious faces, and Vera Iosifovna read her novel. It began like this: "The frost was intense." The windows were wide open; from the kitchen came the clatter of knives and the smell of fried onions. It was comfortable in the soft deep arm chair; the lights had such a friendly twinkle in the twilight of the drawing-room and at the moment on a summer evening when sounds of voices and laughter floated in from the street and whiffs of lilac from the yard, it was difficult to grasp that the frost was intense, and that the setting sun was lighting with its chilly rays a solitary wayfarer on the snowy plain. Vera Iosifovna read how a beautiful young countess founded a school, a hospital, a library, in her village, and fell in love with a wandering artist; she read of what never happens in real life, and yet it was pleasant to listen—it was comfortable, and such agreeable, serene thoughts kept coming into the mind, one had no desire to get up.

"Not bad. ..." Ivan Petrovitch said softly.

And one of the visitors hearing, with his thoughts far away, said hardly audibly: "Yes . . . truly. . . ."

One hour passed, another. In the town gardens close by a band was playing and a chorus was singing. When Vera Iosifovna shut her manuscript book, the company was silent for five minutes, listening to "Lutchina" being sung by the chorus, and the song gave what was not in the novel and is in real life.

"Do you publish your stories in magazines?" Startsev asked Vera Iosifovna.

"No," she answered. "I never publish. I write it and put it away in my cupboard. Why publish?" she explained. "We have enough to live on."

And for some reason everyone sighed.

"And now, Kitten, you play something," Ivan Petrovitch said to his daughter.

The lid of the piano was raised and the music lying ready was opened. Ekaterina Ivanovna sat down and banged on the piano with both hands, and then banged again with all her might, and then again and again; her shoulders and bosom shook. She obstinately banged on the same notes, and it sounded as if she would not leave off until she had hammered the keys into the piano. The drawing-room was filled with the din; everything was resounding; the floor, the ceiling, the furniture. . . . Ekaterina Ivanovna was playing a difficult passage, interesting simply on account of its difficulty, long and monotonous, and Startsev, listening, pictured stones dropping down a steep hill and going on dropping, and he wished they would leave off dropping; and at the same time Ekaterina Ivanovna, rosy from the violent exercise, strong and vigorous, with a lock of hair falling over her forehead, attracted him very much. After the winter spent at Dyalizh among patients and peasants, to sit in a drawing-room, to watch this young, elegant, and, in all probability, pure creature, and to listen to these noisy, tedious but still cultured sounds, was so pleasant, so novel.

"Well, Kitten, you have played as never before," said Ivan Petrovitch, with tears in his eyes, when his daughter had finished and stood up. "Die, Denis; you won't write anything better."

All flocked round her, congratulated her, expressed astonishment, declared that it was long since they had heard such music, and she listened in silence with a faint smile, and her whole figure was expressive of triumph.

"Splendid, superb!"

"Splendid," said Startsev, too, carried away by the general enthusiasm. "Where have you studied?" He asked Ekaterina Ivanovna. "At the Conservatoire?"

"No, I am only preparing for the Conservatoire, and till now have been working with Madame Zavlovsky."

"Have you finished at the high school here?"

"On, no," Vera Iosifovna answered for her. "We have teachers for her at home; there might be bad influences at the high school or a boarding school, you know.

While a young girl is growing up, she ought to be under no influence but her mother's."

"All the same, I'm going to the Conservatoire," said Ekaterina Ivanovna.

"No. Kitten loves her mamma. Kitten won't grieve papa and mamma."

"No, I'm going, I'm going," said Ekaterina Ivanovna, with playful caprice and stamping her foot.

And at supper it was Ivan Petrovitch who displayed his talents. Laughing only with his eyes he told anecdotes, made epigrams, asked ridiculous riddles and answered them himself, talking the whole time in his extraordinary language, evolved in the course of prolonged practice in witticism and evidently now become a habit: "Badsome," "Hugeous," "Thank you most dumbly," and so on.

But that was not all. When the guests, replete and satisfied, trooped into the hall, looking for their coats and sticks, there bustled about them the footman Pavlusha, or, as he was called in the family, Pava—a lad of fourteen with shaven head and chubby cheeks.

"Come, Pava, perform!" Ivan Petrovitch said to him.

Pava struck an attitude, flung up his arm, and said in a tragic tone: "Unhappy woman, die!"

And everyone roared with laughter.

"It's entertaining," thought Startsev, as he went out into the street.

He went to a restaurant and drank some beer, then set off to walk home to Dyalizh; he walked all the way singing.

"'Thy voice to me so languid and caressing . . .'"

On going to bed, he felt not the slightest fatigue after the six miles' walk. On the contrary, he felt as though he could with pleasure have walked another twenty.

"Not badsome," he thought, and laughed as he fell asleep.

II

Startsev kept meaning to go to the Turkins' again, but there was a great deal of work in the hospital, and he was unable to find free time. In this way more than a year passed in work and solitude. But one day a letter in a light blue envelope was brought him from the town.

Vera Iosifovna had been suffering for some time from migraine, but now since Kitten frightened her every day by saying that she was going away to the Conservatoire, the attacks began to be more frequent. All the doctors of the town had been at the Turkins'; at last it was the district doctor's turn. Vera Iosifovna wrote him a touching letter in which she begged him to come and relieve her sufferings. Startsev went, and after that he began to be very often at the Turkins.' He really did something for Vera Iosifovna, and she was already telling all her visitors that he was a wonderful and exceptional doctor. But it was not for the sake of her migraine that he visited the Turkins' now.

It was a holiday. Ekaterina Ivanovna finished her long, wearisome exercise on the piano. Then they sat a long time in the dining-room, drinking tea, and Ivan Petrovitch told some amusing story. Then there was a ring and he had to go into the hall to welcome a guest; Startsev took advantage of the momentary commotion, and whispered to Ekaterina Ivanovna in great agitation:

"For God's sake, I entreat you, don't torment me; let us go into the garden!"

She shrugged her shoulders, as though perplexed and not knowing what he wanted of her, but she got up and went.

"You play the piano for three or four hours," he said, following her; "then you sit with your mother, and there is no possibility of speaking to you. Give me a quarter of an hour at least, I beseech you."

Autumn was approaching, and it was quiet and melancholy in the old garden; the dark leaves lay thick in the walks. It was already beginning to get dark early.

"I haven't seen you for a whole week," Startsev went on, "and if you only knew what suffering it is! Let us sit down. Listen to me."

They had a favorite place in the garden; a seat under an old spreading maple. And now they sat down on this seat.

"What do you want?" said Ekaterina Ivanovna dryly, in a matter-of-fact tone.

"I have not seen you for a whole week; I have not heard you for so long. I long passionately, I thirst for your voice. Speak."

She fascinated him by her freshness, the naïve expression of her eyes and cheeks. Even in the way her dress hung on her, he saw something extraordinarily charming, touching in its simplicity and naïve grace; and at the same time, in spite of this naïveté, she seemed to him intelligent and developed beyond her years. He could talk with her about literature, about art, about anything he liked; could complain to her of life, of people, though it sometimes happened in the middle of serious conversation she would laugh inappropriately or run away into the house. Like almost all girls of her neighborhood, she had a read a great deal (as a rule people read very little in S——, and at the lending library they said if it were not for the girls and the young Jews, they might as well shut up the library). This afforded Startsev infinite delight; he used to ask her eagerly every time what she had been reading the last few days, and listened enthralled while she told him.

"What have you been reading this week since I saw you last?" he asked now. "Do please tell me."

"I have been reading Pisemsky."

"What exactly?"

"'A Thousand Souls,'" answered Kitten. "And what a funny name Pisemsky had—Alexey Feofilaktitch!"

"Where are you going?" cried Startsev in horror, as she suddenly got up and walked towards the house. "I must talk to you; I want to explain myself. Stay with me just five minutes, I supplicate you!"

She stopped as though she wanted to say something, then awkwardly thrust a note into his hand, ran home and sat down to the piano again.

"Be in the cemetery," Startsev read, "at eleven o'clock to-night, near the tomb of Demetti."

"Well, that's not at all clever," he thought, coming to himself. "Why the cemetery? What for?"

It was clear: Kitten was playing a prank. Who would seriously dream of making an appointment at night in the cemetery far out of the town, when it might haven been arranged in the street or in the town gardens? And was it in keeping with him—a district doctor, an intelligent, staid man—to be sighing, receiving notes, to hang about cemeteries, to do silly things that even schoolboys think ridiculous nowadays? What would this romance lead to? What would his colleagues say when they heard of it? Such were Startsev's reflections as he wandered round the tables at the club, and at half past ten he suddenly set off for the cemetery.

By now he had his own pair of horses, and a coachman called Panteleimon, in a velvet waistcoat. The moon was shining. It was still warm, warm as it is in autumn. Dogs were howling in the suburb near the slaughter-house. Startsev left his horses in one of the side-streets at the end of the town, and walked on foot to the cemetery.

"We all have our oddities," he thought. "Kitten is odd, too; and—who knows?— perhaps she is not joking, perhaps she will come"; and he abandoned himself to this faint, vain hope, and it intoxicated him.

He walked for half a mile through fields; the cemetery showed as a dark streak in the distance, like a forest or a big garden. The wall of white stone came into sight, the gate. In the moonlight he could read on the gate: "The hour cometh." Startsev went in at the little gate, and before anything else he saw the white crosses and monuments on both sides of the broad avenue, and the black shadows of them and the poplars; and for a long way round it was all white and black, and the slumbering trees bowed their branches over the white stones. It seemed as though it were lighter here than in the fields; the maple-leaves stood out sharply like paws on the yellow sand of the avenue and on the stones, and the inscriptions on the tombs could be clearly read. For the first moments Startsev was struck now by what he saw for the first time in his life, and what he would probably never see again; a world not like anything else, a world in which the moonlight was as soft and beautiful, as though slumbering here in its cradle, where there was no life, none whatever; but in every dark poplar, in every tomb, there was felt the presence of a mystery that promised a life peaceful, beautiful, eternal. The stones and faded flowers, together with the autumn scent of the leaves, all told of forgiveness, melancholy, and peace.

All was silence around; the stars looked down from the sky in the profound stillness, and Startsev's footsteps sounded loud and out of place, and only when the church clock began striking and he imagined himself dead, buried there forever, he felt as though someone were looking at him, and for a moment he thought that it was not peace and tranquility, but stifled despair, the dumb dreariness of non-existence.

Demitti's tomb was in the form of a shrine with an angel at the top. The Italian opera had once visited S——and one of the singers had died; she had been buried here, and this monument put up to her. No one in the town remembered her, but the lamp at the entrance reflected the moonlight, and looked as though it were burning.

There was no one, and, indeed, who would come here at midnight? But Startsev waited, and as though the moonlight warmed his passion, he waited passionately, and, in imagination, pictured kisses and embraces. He sat near the monument for half an hour, then paced up and down the side avenues, with his hat in his hands, waiting and thinking of the many women and girls buried in these tombs who had been beautiful and fascinating, who had loved, at night burned with passion, yielding themselves to caresses. How wickedly Mother Nature jested at man's expense, after all! How humiliating it was to recognize it!

Startsev thought this, and at the same time he wanted to cry out that he wanted love, that he was eager for it at all costs. To his eyes they were not slabs of marble, but fair white bodies in the moonlight; he saw shapes hiding bashfully in the shadows of the trees, felt their warmth, and the languor was oppressive.

And as though a curtain were lowered, the moon went behind a cloud, and suddenly all was darkness. Startsev could scarcely find the gate—by now it was as dark as it is on an autumn night. Then he wandered about for an hour and a half, looking for the side-street in which he had left his horses.

"I am tired; I can scarcely stand on my legs," he said to Panteleimon.

And settling himself with relief in his carriage, he thought: "Och! I ought not to get fat!"

III

The following evening he went to the Turkins' to make an offer. But it turned out to be an inconvenient moment, as Ekaterina Ivanovna was in her own room having her hair done by a hair dresser. She was getting ready to go to a dance at the club.

He had to sit a long time again in the dining-room drinking tea. Ivan Petrovitch, seeing that his visitor was bored and preoccupied, drew some notes out of his waistcoat pocket, read a funny letter from a German steward, saying that all the ironmongery was ruined and the plasticity was peeling off the walls.

"I expect they will give a decent dowry," thought Startsev, listening absent-mindedly.

After a sleepless night, he found himself in a state of stupefaction, as though he had been given something sweet and soporific to drink; there was fog in his soul, but joy and warmth, and at the same time a sort of cold, heavy fragment of his brain was reflecting:

"Stop before it is too late! Is she the match for you? She is spoilt, whimsical, sleeps till two o'clock in the afternoon, while you are a deacon's son, a district doctor. . . ."

"What of it?" he thought. "I don't care."

"Besides, if you marry her," the fragment went on, "then her relations will make you give up the district work and live in the town."

"After all," he thought, "if it must be the town, the town it must be. They will give a dowry; we can establish ourselves suitably."

At last Ekaterina Ivanovna came in, dressed for the ball, with a low neck, looking fresh and pretty and Startsev admired her so much, and went into such ecstasies, that he could say nothing, but simply stared at her and laughed.

She began saying good-by, and he—he had no reason for staying now—got up, saying that it was time for him to go home: his patients were waiting for him.

"Well, there's no help for that," said Ivan Petrovitch. "Go, and you might take Kitten to the club on the way."

It was spotting with rain; it was very dark, and they could only tell where the horses were by Panteleimon's husky cough. The hood of the carriage was put up.

"I stand upright; you lie down right; he lies all right," said Ivan Petrovitch as he put his daughter into the carriage.

They drove off.

"I was at the cemetery yesterday," Startsev began. "How ungenerous and merciless it was on your part!"

"You went to the cemetery?"

"Yes, I went there and waited almost till two o'clock. I suffered."

"Well, suffer, if you cannot understand a joke."

Ekaterina Ivanovna, pleased at having so cleverly taken in a man who was in love with her, and at being the object of such intense love, burst out laughing and suddenly uttered a shriek of terror for, at that very minute, the horses turned sharply in at the gate of the club, and the carriage almost tilted over. Startsev put his arm round Ekaterina Ivanovna's waist; in her fright she nestled up to him, and he could not restrain himself, and passionately kissed her on the lips and on the chin, and hugged her more tightly.

"That's enough," she said dryly.

And a minute later she was not in the carriage, and a policeman near the lighted entrance of the club shouted in a detestable voice to Panteleimon:

"What are you stopping for, you crow? Drive on."

Startsev drove home, but soon afterwards returned. Attired in another man's dress suit and stiff white tie that kept sawing at his neck and trying to slip away from the collar, he was sitting at midnight in the club drawing-room, and was saying with enthusiasm to Ekaterina Ivanovna:

"Ah, how little people know who have never loved! It seems to me that no one has ever yet written of love truly, and I doubt whether this tender, joyful, agonizing feeling can be described, and anyone who has once experienced it would not attempt to put it into words. What is the use of preliminaries and introductions? What is the use of unnecessary fine words? My love is immeasurable. I beg, I beseech you," Startsev brought out at last, "be my wife!"

"Dmitri Ionitch," said Ekaterina Ivanovna, with a very grave face, after a moment's thought—"Dmitri Ionitch, I am very grateful to you for the honor. I respect you, but . . ." she got up and continued standing, "but, forgive me, I cannot be your wife. Let us talk seriously. Dmitri Ionitch, you know I love art beyond everything in life. I adore music; I love it frantically; I have dedicated my whole life to it. I want to be an artist; I want fame, success, freedom, and you want me to go on living in this town, to go on living this empty, useless life, which has become insufferable to me. To become a wife—oh, no forgive me! One must strive towards a lofty, glorious goal, and married life would put me in bondage forever, Dmitri Ionitch" (She faintly smiled as she pronounced his name; she thought of "Alexey Feofilaktitch")—"Dmitri Ionitch, you are a good, clever, honorable man; you are better than anyone." Tears came into her eyes. "I feel for you with my whole heart, but . . . but you will understand."

And she turned away and went out of the drawing room to prevent herself from crying.

Startsev's heart left off throbbing uneasily. Going out of the club into the street, he first of all tore off the stiff tie and drew a deep breath. He was ashamed and his vanity was wounded (he had not expected a refusal) and could not believe that all his dreams, his hopes and yearnings, had led him up to such a stupid end, just as in some little play at an amateur performance, and he was sorry for his feeling, for that love of his, so sorry that he felt as though he could have burst into sobs or have violently belabored Panteleimon's broad back with his umbrella.

For three days he could not get on with anything, he could not eat nor sleep; but when the news reached him that Ekaterina Ivanovna had gone away to Moscow to enter the Conservatoire, he grew calmer and lived as before.

Afterwards, remembering sometimes how he had wandered about the cemetery or how he had driven all over the town to get a dress suit, he stretched lazily and said:

"What a lot of trouble, though!"

IV

Four years had passed. Startsev already had a large practice in the town. Every morning he hurriedly saw his patients at Dyalizh; then he drove in to see his town patients. By now he drove, not with a pair, but with a team of three with bells on them, and returned home late at night. He had grown broader and stouter, and was not very fond of walking, as he was somewhat asthmatic. And Panteleimon had grown stout, too, and the broader he grew, the more mournfully he sighed and complained of his hard luck: he was sick of driving.

Startsev used to visit various households and met many people, but did not become intimate with anyone. The inhabitants irritated him by their conversation, their views of life, and even their appearance. Experience taught him by degrees that while he played cards or lunched with one of these people, the man was a peaceable, friendly, and even intelligent human being; that as soon as one talked of anything not eatable, for instance, of politics or science, he would be completely at a loss, or would expound philosophy so stupid and ill-natured that there was nothing else to do but wave one's hand in despair and go away. Even when Startsev tried to talk to liberal citizens, saying for instance, that humanity, thank God, was progressing, and that one day it would be possible to dispense with passports and capital punishment, the liberal citizen would look at him askance and ask him mistrustfully: "Then any one could murder anyone he chose in the open street?" And when, at tea or supper, Startsev observed in company that one should work, and that one ought not to live without working, everyone took this as a reproach, and began to get angry and argue aggressively. With all that, the inhabitants did nothing, absolutely nothing, and took no interest in anything, and it was quite impossible to think of anything to say. And Startsev avoided conversation, and confined himself to eating and playing *vint;* and when there was a family festivity in some household and he was invited to a meal, then he sat and ate in silence, looking at his plate. And everything that was said at the time was uninteresting, unjust, and stupid; he felt irritated and disturbed, but held his tongue, and, because he sat glumly silent and looked at his plate, he was nicknamed in the town "the haughty Pole," though he never had been a Pole.

All such entertainments as theatres and concerts he declined, but he played *vint* every evening for three hours with enjoyment. He had another diversion to which he took imperceptibly, little by little: in the evening he would take out of his pockets the notes he had gained by his practice, and sometimes there were stuffed in his pockets notes—yellow and green, and smelling of scent and vinegar and incense and fish oil—up to the value of seventy rubles; and when they amounted to some hundreds he took them to the Mutual Credit Bank and deposited the money there to his account.

He was only twice at the Turkins' in the course of the four years after Ekaterina Ivanovna had gone away, on each occasion at the invitation of Vera Iosifovna, who was still undergoing treatment for migraine. Every summer Ekaterina Ivanovna came to stay with her parents, but he did not once see her; it somehow never happened.

But now four years had passed. One still, warm morning a letter was brought to the hospital. Vera Iosifovna wrote to Dmitri Ionitch that she was missing him very much, and begged him to come and see them, and to relieve her sufferings; and, by the way, it was her birthday. Below was a postscript: "I join in mother's request.—K."

Startsev considered, and in the evening he went to the Turkins'.

"How do you do, if you please?" Ivan Petrovitch met him, smiling with his eyes only. "Bonjour."

Vera Iosifovna, white-haired and looking much older, shook Startsev's hand, sighed affectedly, and said:

"You don't care to pay attention to me, doctor. You never come and see us; I am too old for you. But now someone young has come; perhaps she will be more fortunate."

And Kitten? She had grown thinner, paler, had grown handsomer and more graceful; but now she was Ekaterina Ivanovna, not Kitten; she had lost the freshness and look of childish naïveté. And in her expression and manners there was something new—guilty and diffident, as though she did not feel herself at home here in the Turkins' house.

"How many summers, how many winters!" she said, giving Startsev her hand, and he could see that her heart was beating with excitement; and looking at him intently and curiously, she went on: "How much stouter you are! You look sun burnt and more manly, but on the whole you have changed very little."

Now, too, he thought her attractive, very attractive, but there was something lacking in her, or else something superfluous—he could not himself have said exactly what it was, but something prevented him from feeling as before. He did not like her pallor, her new expression, her faint smile, her voice and soon afterwards he disliked her clothes, too, and the low chair in which she was sitting; he disliked something in the past when he had almost married her. He thought of his love, of the dreams and the hopes that had troubled him four years before— and he felt awkward.

They had tea with cakes. Then Vera Iosifovna read aloud a novel; she read of things that never happen in real life, and Startsev listened, looked at her handsome gray head, and waited for her to finish.

"People are not stupid because they can't write novels, but because they can't conceal it when they do," he thought.

"Not badsome," said Ivan Petrovitch.

Then Ekaterina Ivanovna played long and noisily on the piano, and when she was finished she was profusely thanked and warmly praised.

"It's a good thing I did not marry her," thought Startsev.

She looked at him, and evidently expected him to ask her to go into the garden, but he remained silent.

"Let us have a talk," she said, going up to him. "How are you getting on? What are you doing? How are things? I have been thinking about you all these days," she went on nervously. "I wanted to write to you, wanted to come myself to see you at Dyalizh. I quite made up my mind to go, but afterwards I thought better of it. God knows what your attitude is towards me now; I have been looking forward to seeing you today with such emotion. For goodness' sake let us go into the garden."

They went into the garden and sat down on the seat under the old maple, just as they had done four years before. It was dark.

"How are you getting on?" asked Ekaterina Ivanovna.

"Oh, all right; I am jogging along," answered Startsev.

And he could think of nothing more. They were silent.

"I feel so excited!" said Ekaterina Ivanovna, and she hid her face in her hands. "But don't pay attention to it. I am so happy to be at home; I am so glad to see everyone. I can't get used to it. So many memories! I thought we should talk without stopping till morning."

Now he saw her face near, her shining eyes, and in the darkness she looked younger than in the room, and even her old childish expression seemed to have come back to her. And indeed she was looking at him with naïve curiosity, as though she wanted to get a closer view and understanding of the man who had loved her so ardently, with such tenderness, and so unsuccessfully; her eyes thanked him for that love. And he remembered all that had been, every minute detail; how he had wandered about the cemetery, how he had returned home in the morning exhausted, and he suddenly felt sad and regretted the past. A warmth began glowing in his heart.

"Do you remember how I took you to the dance at the club?" he asked. "It was dark and rainy. . . ."

The warmth was glowing now in his heart, and he longed to talk, to rail at life.

"Ech!" he said with a sigh. "You ask how I am living. How do we live here? Why, not at all. We grow old, we grow stout, we grow slack. Day after day passes;

life slips by without color, without expressions, without thoughts. In the day-time working for gain, and in the evening the club, the company of card play-ers, alcoholic, raucous-voiced gentlemen whom I can't endure. What is there nice in it?"

"Well, you have work—a noble object in life. You used to be so fond of talking of your hospital. I was such a queer girl then; I imagined myself such a great pia-nist. Nowadays all young ladies play the piano, and I played, too, like everybody else and there was nothing special about me. I am just such a pianist as my mother is an authoress. And of course I didn't understand you then, but afterwards in Moscow I often thought of you. I thought of no one but you. What happiness to be a district doctor; to help the suffering; to be serving the people! What happi-ness!" Ekaterina Ivanovna repeated with enthusiasm. "When I thought of you in Moscow, you seemed to me so ideal, so lofty."

Startsev thought of the notes he used to take out of his pockets in the evening with such pleasure, and the glow in his heart was quenched.

He got up to go into the house. She took his arm.

"You are the best man I've known in my life," she went on. "We will see each other and talk, won't we? Promise me. I am not a pianist; I am not in error about myself now, and I will not play before you or talk of music."

When they had gone into the house, and when Startsev saw in the lamplight her face, and her sad, grateful, searching eyes fixed upon him, he felt uneasy and thought again:

"It's a good thing I did not marry her then."

He began taking leave.

"You have no human right to go before supper," said Ivan Petrovitch as he saw him off. "It's extremely perpendicular on your part. Well, now, perform!" he added, addressing Pava in the hall.

Pava, no longer a boy, but a young man with moustaches, threw himself into an attitude, flung up his arm, and said in a tragic voice:

"Unhappy woman, die!"

All this irritated Startsev. Getting into his carriage, and looking at the dark house and garden which had once been so precious and so dear, he thought of everything at once—Vera Iosifovna's novels and Kitten's noisy playing, and Ivan Petrovitch's jokes and Pava's tragic posturing, and thought if the most talented people in the town were so futile, what must the town be.

Three days later Pava brought a letter from Ekaterina Ivanovna.

"You don't come and see us—why?" she wrote to him. "I am afraid that you have changed towards us. I am afraid, and I am terrified at the very thought of it. Reassure me; come and tell me that everything is well.

"I must talk to you.—Your E. I."

He read this letter, thought a moment, and said to Pava:

"Tell them, my good fellow, that I can't come today; I am very busy. Say I will come in three days or so."

But three days passed, a week passed; he still did not go. Happening once to drive past the Turkins' house, he thought he must go in, if only for a moment, but on second thought . . . did not go in.

And he never went to the Turkins' again.

V

Several more years have passed. Startsev has grown stouter still, has grown corpulent, breathes heavily, and already walks with his head thrown back. When stout and red in the face, he drives with his bells and his team of three horses, and Panteleimon, also stout and red in the face with his thick beefy neck, sits on the box holding his arms stiffly out before him as though they were made of wood, and shouts to those he meets: "Keep to the ri-i-ight!" It is an impressive picture; one might think it was not a mortal but some heathen deity in his chariot. He has an immense practice in the town, not time to breathe, and already has an estate and two houses in the town, and he is looking out for a third more profitable; and when at the Mutual Credit Bank he is told of a house that is for sale, he goes to the house without ceremony, and, marching through all the rooms, regardless of half-dressed women and children who gaze at him in amazement and alarm, he prods at the doors with his stick, and says:

"Is that the study? Is that a bedroom? And what's here?"

And as he does so he breathes heavily and wipes the sweat from his brow.

He has a great deal to do, but still he does not give up his work as district doctor; he is greedy for gain, and he tries to be in all places at once. At Dyalizh and in the town he is called simply "Ionitch": "Where is Ionitch off to?" or "Should not we call in Ionitch to a consultation?"

Probably because his throat is covered with rolls of fat, his voice has changed; it has become thin and sharp. His temper has changed too: he has grown ill-humored and irritable. When he sees his patients he is usually out of temper; he impatiently taps the floor with his stick, and shouts in his disagreeable voice:

"Be so good as to confine yourself to answering my questions! Don't talk so much!"

He is solitary. He leads a dreary life; nothing interests him.

During all the years he had lived at Dyalizh his love for Kitten had been his one joy, and probably his last. In the evenings he plays *vint* at the club, and then sits alone at a big table and has supper. Ivan, the oldest and most respectable of the waiters, serves him, hands him Lafitte No. 17, and every one at the club—

members of the committee, the cook and waiters—know what he likes and what he doesn't like and do their very utmost to satisfy him, or else he is sure to fly into a rage and bang on the floor with his stick.

As he eats his supper, he turns round from time to time and puts in his spoke in some conversation:

"What are you talking about? Eh? Whom?"

And when at a neighboring table there is talk of the Turkins, he asks:

"What Turkins are you speaking of? Do you mean the people whose daughter plays on the piano?"

That is all that can be said about him.

And the Turkins? Ivan Petrovitch has grown no older; he is not changed in the least, and still makes jokes and tells anecdotes as of old. Vera Iosifovna still reads her novels aloud to her visitors with eagerness and touching simplicity. And Kitten plays the piano for four hours every day. She has grown visibly older, is constantly ailing, and every autumn goes to the Crimea with her mother. When Ivan Petrovitch sees them off at the station, he wipes his tears as the train starts, and shouts:

"Good-bye, if you please."

And he waves his handkerchief.

A Doctor's Visit

The Professor received a telegram from the Lyalikovs' factory; he was asked to come as quickly as possible. The daughter of some Madame Lyalikov, apparently the owner of the factory, was ill, and that was all that one could make out of the long, incoherent telegram. And the Professor did not go himself, but sent instead his assistant, Korolyov.

It was two stations from Moscow, and there was a drive of three miles from the station. A carriage with three horses had been sent to the station to meet Korolyov; the coachman wore a hat with a peacock's feather on it, and answered every question in a loud voice like a soldier: "No, sir!" "Certainly, sir!"

It was Saturday evening; the sun was setting, the workpeople were coming in crowds from the factory to the station, and they bowed to the carriage in which Korolyov was driving. And he was charmed with the evening, the farmhouses and villas on the road, and the birch-trees, and the quiet atmosphere all around, when the fields and woods and the sun seemed preparing, like the workpeople now on the eve of the holiday, to rest, and perhaps to pray. . . .

He was born and had grown up in Moscow; he did not know the country, and he had never taken any interest in factories, or been inside one, but he had happened to read about factories, and had been in the houses of manufacturers and had talked to them; and whenever he saw a factory far or near, he always thought how quiet and peaceable it was outside, but within there was always sure to be impenetrable ignorance and dull egoism on the side of the owners, wearisome, unhealthy toil on the side of the workpeople, squabbling, vermin, vodka. And now when the workpeople timidly and respectfully made way for the carriage, in their faces, their caps, their walk, he read physical impurity, drunkenness, nervous exhaustion, bewilderment.

They drove in at the factory gates. On each side he caught glimpses of the little houses of workpeople, of the faces of women, of quilts and linen on the railings. "Look out!" shouted the coachman, not pulling up the horses. It was a wide courtyard without grass, with five immense blocks of buildings with tall chimneys a little distance one from another, warehouses and barracks, and over everything a sort of grey powder as though from dust. Here and there, like oases in the desert, there were pitiful gardens, and the green and red roofs of the houses in which the managers and clerks lived. The coachman suddenly pulled up the horses, and the carriage stopped at the house, which had been newly painted grey; here was a flower garden, with a lilac bush covered with dust, and on the yellow steps at the front door there was a strong smell of paint.

"Please come in, doctor," said women's voices in the passage and the entry, and at the same time he heard sighs and whisperings. "Pray walk in. . . . We've been expecting you so long; we're in real trouble. Here, this way."

Madame Lyalikov—a stout elderly lady wearing a black silk dress with fashionable sleeves, but, judging from her face, a simple uneducated woman—looked at the doctor in a flutter, and could not bring herself to hold out her hand to him; she did not dare. Beside her stood a personage with short hair and a pince-nez; she was wearing a blouse of many colors, and was very thin and no longer young. The servants called her Christina Dmitryevna, and Korolyov guessed that this was the governess. Probably, as the person of most education in the house, she had been charged to meet and receive the doctor, for she began immediately, in great haste, stating the causes of the illness, giving trivial and tiresome details, but without saying who was ill or what was the matter.

The doctor and the governess were sitting talking while the lady of the house stood motionless at the door, waiting. From the conversation Korolyov learned that the patient was Madame Lyalikov's only daughter and heiress, a girl of twenty, called Liza; she had been ill for a long time, and had consulted various doctors, and the previous night she had suffered till morning from such violent palpitations of the heart, that no one in the house had slept, and they had been afraid she might die.

"She has been, one may say, ailing from a child," said Christina Dmitryevna in a sing-song voice, continually wiping her lips with her hand. "The doctors say it is nerves; when she was a little girl she was scrofulous, and the doctors drove it inwards, so I think it may be due to that."

They went to see the invalid. Fully grown up, big and tall, but ugly like her mother, with the same little eyes and disproportionate breadth of the lower part of the face, lying with her hair in disorder, muffled up to the chin, she made upon Korolyov at the first minute the impression of a poor, destitute creature, sheltered and cared for here out of charity, and he could hardly believe that this was the heiress of the five huge buildings.

"I am the doctor come to see you," said Korolyov. "Good evening."

He mentioned his name and pressed her hand, a large, cold, ugly hand; she sat up, and, evidently accustomed to doctors, let herself be sounded, without showing the least concern that her shoulders and chest were uncovered.

"I have palpitations of the heart," she said. "It was so awful all night. . . . I almost died of fright! Do give me something."

"I will, I will; don't worry yourself."

Korolyov examined her and shrugged his shoulders.

"The heart is all right," he said; "it's all going on satisfactorily; everything is in good order. Your nerves must have been playing pranks a little, but that's so common. The attack is over by now, one must suppose; lie down and go to sleep."

At that moment a lamp was brought into the bedroom. The patient screwed up her eyes at the light, then suddenly put her hands to her head and broke into sobs. And the impression of a destitute, ugly creature vanished, and Korolyov no longer noticed the little eyes or the heavy development of the lower part of the face. He saw a soft, suffering expression, which was intelligent and touching: she seemed to him altogether graceful, feminine, and simple; and he longed to soothe her, not with drugs, not with advice, but with simple, kindly words. Her mother put her arms round her head and hugged her. What despair, what grief was in the old woman's face! She, her mother, had reared her and brought her up, spared nothing, and devoted her whole life to having her daughter taught French, dancing, music: had engaged a dozen teachers for her; had consulted the best doctors, kept a governess. And now she could not make out the reason of these tears, why there was all this misery, she could not understand, and was bewildered; and she had a guilty, agitated, despairing expression, as though she had omitted something very important, had left something undone, had neglected to call in somebody—and whom, she did not know.

"Lizanka, you are crying again . . . again," she said, hugging her daughter to her. "My own, my darling, my child, tell me what it is! Have pity on me! Tell me."

Both wept bitterly. Korolyov sat down on the side of the bed and took Liza's hand.

"Come, give over; it's no use crying," he said kindly. "Why, there is nothing in the world that is worth those tears. Come, we won't cry; that's no good."

And inwardly he thought:

"It's high time she was married."

"Our doctor at the factory gave her kalibromati," said the governess, "but I notice it only makes her worse. I should have thought that if she is given anything for the heart it ought to be drops. I forget the name. . . . Convallaria, isn't it?"

And there followed all sorts of details. She interrupted the doctor, preventing his speaking, and there was a look of effort on her face, as though she supposed that, as the woman of most education in the house, she was duty bound to keep up a conversation with the doctor, and on no other subject but medicine.

Korolyov felt bored.

"I find nothing special the matter," he said, addressing the mother as he went out of the bedroom. "If your daughter is being attended by the factory doctor, let him go on attending her. The treatment so far has been perfectly correct, and I see no reason for changing your doctor. Why change? It's such an ordinary trouble; there's nothing seriously wrong."

He spoke deliberately as he put on his gloves, while Madame Lyalikov stood without moving, and looked at him with her tearful eyes.

"I have half an hour to catch the ten o'clock train," he said. "I hope I am not too late."

"And can't you stay?" she asked, and tears trickled down her cheeks again. "I am ashamed to trouble you, but if you would be so good. . . . For God's sake," she went on in an undertone, glancing towards the door, "do stay to-night with us! She is all I have . . . my only daughter. . . . She frightened me last night; I can't get over it. . . . Don't go away, for goodness' sake!"

He wanted to tell her that he had a great deal of work in Moscow, that his family were expecting him home; it was disagreeable to him to spend the evening and the whole night in a strange house quite needlessly; but he looked at her face, heaved a sigh, and began taking off his gloves without a word.

All the lamps and candles were lighted in his honor in the drawing-room and the dining-room. He sat down at the piano and began turning over the music. Then he looked at the pictures on the walls, at the portraits. The pictures, oil-paintings in gold frames, were views of the Crimea—a stormy sea with a ship, a Catholic monk with a wineglass; they were all dull, smooth daubs, with no trace of talent in them. There was not a single good-looking face among the portraits, nothing but broad cheekbones and astonished-looking eyes. Lyalikov, Liza's father, had a low forehead and a self-satisfied expression; his uniform sat like a sack on his bulky plebeian figure; on his breast was a medal and a Red Cross Badge. There was little sign of culture, and the luxury was senseless and haphazard, and was as ill-fitting as that uniform. The floors irritated him with their brilliant polish, the lusters on the chandelier irritated him, and he was reminded for some reason of the story of the merchant who used to go to the baths with a medal on his neck.

He heard a whispering in the entry; someone was softly snoring. And suddenly from outside came harsh, abrupt, metallic sounds, such as Korolyov had never heard before, and which he did not understand now; they roused strange, unpleasant echoes in his soul.

"I believe nothing would induce me to remain here to live," he thought, and went back to the music-books again.

"Doctor, please come to supper!" the governess called him in a low voice.

He went into supper. The table was large and laid with vast number of dishes and wines, but there were only two to supper: himself and Christina Dmitryevna. She drank Madeira, ate rapidly, and talked, looking at him through her pince-nez:

"Our workpeople are very contented. We have performances at the factory every winter; the workpeople act themselves. They have lectures with a magic lantern, a splendid tea-room, and everything they want. They are very much attached to us, and when they heard that Lizanka was worse they had a service sung for her. Though they have no education, they have their feelings, too."

"It looks as though you have no man in the house at all," said Korolyov.

"Not one. Pyotr Nikanoritch died a year and a half ago, and left us alone. And so there are the three of us. In the summer we live here, and in winter we live in Moscow, in Polianka. I have been living with them for eleven years—as one of the family."

At supper they served sterlet, chicken rissoles, and stewed fruit; the wines were expensive French wines.

"Please don't stand on ceremony, doctor," said Christina Dmitryevna, eating and wiping her mouth with her fist, and it was evident she found her life here exceedingly pleasant. "Please have some more."

After supper the doctor was shown to his room, where a bed had been made up for him, but he did not feel sleepy. The room was stuffy and it smelt of paint; he put on his coat and went out.

It was cool in the open air; there was already a glimmer of dawn, and all the five blocks of buildings, with their tall chimneys, barracks, and warehouses, were distinctly outlined against the damp air. As it was a holiday, they were not working, and the windows were dark, and in only one of the buildings was there a furnace burning; two windows were crimson, and fire mixed with smoke came from time to time from the chimney. Far away beyond the yard the frogs were croaking and the nightingales singing.

Looking at the factory buildings and the barracks, where the workpeople were asleep, he thought again what he always thought when he saw a factory. They may have performances for the workpeople, magic lanterns, factory doctors, and improvements of all sorts, but, all the same, the workpeople he had met that day on his way from the station did not look in any way different from those he had known long ago in his childhood, before there were factory performances and improvements. As a doctor accustomed to judging correctly of chronic complaints, the radical cause of which was incomprehensible and incurable, he looked upon factories as something baffling, the cause of which also was obscure and not removable, and all the improvements in the life of the factory hands he looked upon not as superfluous, but as comparable with the treatment of incurable illnesses.

"There is something baffling in it, of course," he thought, looking at the crimson windows. "Fifteen hundred or two thousand workpeople are working without rest in unhealthy surroundings, making bad cotton goods, living on the verge of starvation, and only waking from this nightmare at rare intervals in the tavern; a hundred people act as overseers, and the whole life of that hundred is spent in imposing fines, in abuse, in injustice, and only two or three so-called owners enjoy the profits, though they don't work at all, and despise the wretched cotton. But what are the profits, and how do they enjoy them? Madame Lyalikov and her daughter are unhappy—it makes one wretched to look at them; the only one who enjoys her life is Christina Dmitryevna, a stupid, middle-aged maiden lady in pince-nez. And so it appears that all these five blocks of buildings are at work, and inferior cotton is sold in the Eastern markets, simply that Christina Dmitryevna may eat sterlet and drink Madeira."

Suddenly there came a strange noise, the same sound Korolyov had heard before supper. Some one was striking on a sheet of metal near one of the buildings; he struck a note, and then at once checked the vibrations, so that short, abrupt, discordant sounds were produced, rather like "Dair . . . dair . . . dair. . . ." Then there was half a minute of stillness, and from another building there came sounds equally abrupt and unpleasant, lower bass notes: "Drin . . . drin . . . drin." Eleven times. Evidently it was the watchman striking the hour.

Near the third building he heard: "Zhuk . . . zhuk . . . zhuk. . . ." And so near all the buildings, and then behind the barracks and beyond the gates. And in the stillness of the night it seemed as though these sounds were uttered by a monster with crimson eyes—the devil himself, who controlled the owners and the workpeople alike, and was deceiving both.

Korolyov went out of the yard into the open country.

"Who goes there?" someone called to him at the gates in an abrupt voice.

"It's just like being in prison," he thought, and made no answer.

Here the nightingales and the frogs could be heard more distinctly, and one could feel it was a night in May. From the station came the noise of a train; somewhere in the distance drowsy cocks were crowing; but, all the same, the night was still, the world was sleeping tranquilly. In a field not far from the factory there could be seen the framework of a house and heaps of building material: Korolyov sat down on the planks and went on thinking.

"The only person who feels happy here is the governess, and the factory hands are working for her gratification. But that's only apparent: she is only the figurehead. The real person, for whom everything is being done, is the devil."

And he thought about the devil, in whom he did not believe, and he looked round at the two windows where the fires were gleaming. It seemed to him that out of those crimson eyes the devil himself was looking at him—that unknown force that had created the mutual relation of the strong and the weak, that coarse blunder which one could never correct. The strong must hinder the weak from living—such was the law of Nature; but only in a newspaper article or in a schoolbook was that intelligible and easily accepted. In the hotchpotch which was everyday life, in the tangle of trivialities out of which human relations were woven, it was no longer a law, but a logical absurdity, when the strong and the weak were both equally victims of their mutual relations, unwillingly submitting to some directing force, unknown, standing outside life, apart from man.

So thought Korolyov, sitting on the planks, and little by little he was possessed by a feeling that this unknown and mysterious force was really close by and looking at him. Meanwhile the east was growing paler, time passed rapidly; when there was not a soul anywhere near, as though everything were dead, the five buildings and their chimneys against the grey background of the dawn had a peculiar look—not the same as by day; one forgot altogether that inside there were steam motors, electricity, telephones, and kept thinking of lake-dwellings, of the Stone Age, feeling the presence of a crude, unconscious force. . . .

And again there came the sound: "Dair . . . dair . . . dair . . . dair" . . . twelve times.

Then there was stillness, stillness for half a minute, and at the other end of the yard there rang out.

Drin . . . drin . . . drin.

"Horribly disagreeable," thought Korolyov.

"Zhuk . . . zhuk . . ." there resounded from a third place, abruptly, sharply, as though with annoyance—"Zhuk . . . zhuk . . ."

And it took four minutes to strike twelve. Then there was a hush; and again it seemed as though everything were dead.

Korolyov sat a little longer, then went to the house, but sat up for a good while longer. In the adjoining rooms there was whispering, there was a sound of shuffling slippers and bare feet.

"Is she having another attack?" thought Korolyov.

He went out to have a look at the patient. By now it was quite light in the rooms, and a faint glimmer of sunlight, piercing through the morning mist, quivered on the floor and on the wall of the drawing-room. The door of Liza's room was open, and she was sitting in a low chair beside her bed, with her hair down, wearing a dressing-gown and wrapped in a shawl. The blinds were down on the windows.

"How do you feel?" asked Korolyov.

"Thank you."

He touched her pulse, then straightened her hair, that had fallen over her forehead.

"You are not asleep," he said. "It's beautiful weather outside. It's spring. The nightingales are singing, and you sit in the dark and think of something."

She listened and looked into his face; her eyes were sorrowful and intelligent, and it was evident she wanted to say something to him.

"Does this happen to you often?" he said.

She moved her lips, and answered:

"Often, I feel wretched almost every night."

At that moment the watchman in the yard began striking two o'clock. They heard: "Dair . . . dair . . ." and she shuddered.

"Do those knockings worry you?" he asked.

"I don't know. Everything here worries me," she answered, and pondered. "Everything worries me. I hear sympathy in your voice; it seemed to me as soon as I saw you that I could tell you all about it."

"Tell me, I beg you."

"I want to tell you of my opinion. It seems to me that I have no illness, but that I am weary and frightened, because it is bound to be so and cannot be otherwise. Even the healthiest person can't help being uneasy if, for instance, a robber is moving about under his window. I am constantly being doctored," she went on, looking at her knees, and she gave a shy smile. "I am very grateful, of course, and I do not deny that the treatment is a benefit; but I should like to talk, not with a doctor, but with some intimate friend who would understand me and would convince me that I was right or wrong."

"Have you no friends?" asked Korolyov.

"I am lonely. I have a mother; I love her, but, all the same, I am lonely. That's how it happens to be. . . . Lonely people read a great deal, but say little and hear little. Life for them is mysterious; they are mystics and often see the devil where he is not. Lermontov's Tamara was lonely and she saw the devil."

"Do you read a great deal?"

"Yes. You see, my whole time is free from morning till night. I read by day, and by night my head is empty; instead of thoughts there are shadows in it."

"Do you see anything at night? " asked Korolyov.

"No, but I feel . . ."

She smiled again, raised her eyes to the doctor, and looked at him so sorrowfully, so intelligently; and it seemed to him that she trusted him, and that she wanted to speak frankly to him, and that she thought the same as he did. But she was silent, perhaps waiting for him to speak.

And he knew what to say to her. It was clear to him that she needed as quickly as possible to give up the five buildings and the million if she had it—to leave that devil that looked out at night; it was clear to him, too, that she thought so herself, and was only waiting for some one she trusted to confirm her.

But he did not know how to say it. How? One is shy of asking men under sentence what they have been sentenced for; and in the same way it is awkward to ask very rich people what they want so much money for, why they make such a poor use of their wealth, why they don't give it up, even when they see in it their unhappiness; and if they begin a conversation about it themselves, it is usually embarrassing, awkward, and long.

"How is one to say it?" Korolyov wondered. "And is it necessary to speak?"

And he said what he meant in a roundabout way:

"You in the position of a factory owner and a wealthy heiress are dissatisfied; you don't believe in your right to it; and here now you can't sleep. That, of course, is better than if you were satisfied, slept soundly, and thought everything was satisfactory. Your sleeplessness does you credit; in any case, it is a good sign. In reality, such a conversation as this between us now would have been unthinkable for our parents. At night they did not talk, but slept sound; we, our generation, sleep badly, are restless, but talk a great deal, and are always trying to settle whether we are right or not. For our children or grandchildren that question whether they are right or not—will have been settled. Things will be clearer for them than for us. Life will be good in fifty years' time; it's only a pity we shall not last out till then. It would be interesting to have a peep at it."

"What will our children and grandchildren do?" asked Liza.

"I don't know. . . . I suppose they will throw it all up and go away."

"Go where?"

"Where? . . . Why, where they like," said Korolyov; and he laughed. "There are lots of places a good, intelligent person can go to."

He glanced at his watch.

"The sun has risen, though," he said. "It is time you were asleep. Undress and sleep soundly. Very glad to have made your acquaintance," he went on, pressing her hand. "You are a good, interesting woman. Good-night!"

He went to his room and went to bed.

In the morning when the carriage was brought round they all came out on to the steps to see him off. Liza, pale and exhausted, was in a white dress as though for a holiday, with a flower in her hair; she looked at him, as yesterday, sorrowfully and intelligently, smiled and talked, and all with an expression as though she wanted to tell him something special, important—him alone. They could hear the larks trilling and the church bells pealing. The windows in the factory buildings were sparkling gaily, and, driving across the yard and afterwards along the road to the station, Korolyov thought neither of the workpeople nor of lake dwellings, nor of the devil, but thought of the time, perhaps close at hand, when life would be as bright and joyous as that still Sunday morning; and he thought how pleasant it was on such a morning in the spring to drive with three horses in a good carriage, and to bask in the sunshine.

Comments on Chekhov's Doctors

೪

In the following comments, I present a few of my own reflections on these characters and their stories. I'd love to be able to sit down and discuss them with Chekhov himself, to learn what he really thought about these doctors, and whether my diagnoses are correct. The universe being what it is, that appears to be impossible. Thus, these are just the thoughts of one passionate reader.

INTRIGUES

In "Intrigues" (1883) the medical student writer takes a comic view of a puffed-up senior physician whom he might have encountered on his rounds in the hospital, or at the University of Moscow Medical School. Chekhov's Dr. Shelestov is pompous and vainglorious, a big shot whose professional opinion is worth its weight in . . . well, in floating kidneys. Shelestov is outraged because a colleague has accused him of mishandling the affair of October 2. How could he, the great Shelestov, be negligent? What an unthinkable idea!

Chekhov had fine role models in medical school. One was Dr. Grigory Zakharin, his professor of medicine, who had brought the latest European scientific and clinical developments to Moscow. Another was Dr. Eric Erismann, professor of public health, who was later fired from his prestigious job because of his support for a group of student political activists. A third mentor was Dr. Aleksei Ostromov, whom fifteen years later Chekhov would choose as his own doctor when he had a massive lung hemorrhage in 1897.

However, human nature being what it is, the young Chekhov must also have encountered plenty of Shelestov-like physicians as well, doctors chock full of bluster and fuzzy theories. In this sketch Shelestov stands before a mirror, preparing to confront his accusers. With his reputation threatened and his job hanging in the balance, he has to put on a good show. He fantasizes the outcome. Not only will he prove his innocence, but also he will be so impressive that his colleagues will stand and cheer. They will censure Shelestov's opponents. They will elect him president of the medical association. With his enemies smashed, the great Shelestov will bask in universal admiration.

The only problem is that Shelestov can't square these fantasies with the furtive, weasel-like image that stares back at him from the mirror. In medicine, as in all of life, self-deception abounds.

MALINGERERS

In "Malingerers" (1885) we meet Marfa Petrovna Petchonkin, a beloved homeopathic physician. One middle-aged patient had suffered for eight years from rheumatism while other doctors "did me nothing but harm." "All they care about is their fees, the brigands; but as for the benefit of the community—for that they don't care a straw." Allopathic physicians prescribe pills and potions, but they never get to the root of the problem. Rather, they just suppress the symptoms. Worse yet, they may complicate the problem by treating too aggressively. Not so, however, with Dr. Petchonkin, who pursues a simple and gentle homeopathic philosophy.

But perhaps her success stems from something other than homeopathic remedies. Marfa seems to understand that much of her power arises from factors like the natural history of the disease, or the healing influence of her concern (what we would today call the placebo effect). Dr. Petchonkin believes that allopathic medical treatments are ineffective and even harmful, a view shared at least in part by her creator, who tended to be skeptical about the value of contemporary "scientific" therapies, especially for tuberculosis.

Dr. Petchonkin thrives on her patients' gratitude. She not only "cures" them, but also provides them with gifts and favors, like offering to pay for a patient's daughter's education. In all this Marfa demonstrates an intuitive perception of the connection between care and healing. Her level of nurturing seems to move beyond the bounds of medical professionalism. Emotional attachment may rob her of clinical distance and objectivity. Yet Marfa at least preserves enough objectivity to step back from the situation and wonder about the source of her healing power, a step that many scientific doctors never take.

Marfa's compassionate attitude returns as an element in some of the more complex physician characters that appear later in Chekhov's oeuvre; for example, Dymov ("The Grasshopper," 1892), Samoylenko ("The Duel," 1892), and especially, Korolyov ("A Doctor's Visit," 1898).

EXCELLENT PEOPLE

"Excellent People" (1886) poses a question that unsettles the whole essence of medicine. What good is it to fight disease and postpone death? Why not simply accept the world as it is? What difference do we make?

Chekhov puts these sentiments into the mouth of Vera, a female doctor whose husband died of typhus shortly after their marriage, who later survived a suicide attempt. Now she lives with her brother. All she seems to do is mope around and speak mournfully about the failure of civilization. She believes society is corrupt, and science is arrogant and empty. Science will never make the world a better place to live.

Vera's ideas are meant to communicate (or caricature) those of Leo Tolstoy, who was at that time Russia's greatest and most beloved writer. The much younger Chekhov admired Tolstoy as a person but rejected most of the older man's social and moral ideas, including the concept of passive resistance to evil, a religious philosophy that Mohandas Gandhi and Martin Luther King were later to adapt and develop in a much more socially constructive manner. In his own life, Chekhov avoided large-scale social movements or political action, but he also rejected Tolstoy's religious passivity. Instead, he believed in direct action by individuals. In essence, he modeled a "case-based" approach in which each person does what he or she can to remedy specific problems, rather than wasting energy debating the "big picture."

Vera's brother and his friends are bored with her incessant doom saying. They pity her but wish she would simply go away. Inexplicably, one day Vera undergoes a conversion. She activates herself, announcing that she intends to become a public health doctor in the provinces and work for the betterment of society. What happens then? Does she meet with success? Does she lead a fulfilling life? The reader is left to decide.

ANYUTA

In "Anyuta" (1886) a medical student is studying anatomy, while his live-in concubine sits across the room, shivering and mending his clothes. It is freezing. Times are tough. They can't afford to buy fuel to heat the flat. Suddenly, the student demands that Anyuta remove her blouse so that she can serve as an anatomical model. She complies. Shortly thereafter, an artist who lives in the same building drops in to request that Anyuta come down to his studio to pose in the nude. Once again, she willingly complies.

The medical student approaches Anyuta with scientific objectivity. He delineates the parameters of her body, which is, after all, merely a container of bones and organs. The woman is an animated textbook, a means of cramming for the exam. This sort of insensitivity is not the exclusive province of science. Fedisov, the artist, also objectifies the young woman. He views her from the aesthetic perspective—lines, curves, color, and the image of beauty she embodies. Neither of these callow young men connects with her as a person. Neither approaches her with warmth or compassion. They abuse her with their cold and calculating stares.

THE DOCTOR

Dr. Tsvyetkov in "The Doctor" (1886) experiences the dilemma of conflicting personal and professional roles. We find him sitting at the bedside of a small boy dying of a brain tumor. In the next room, the boy's mother sits, grieving. The complicating factor is that Dr. Tsvyetkov once had an affair with the boy's unmarried mother, who has always told Tsvyetkov that Misha is his son.

Now that Misha lies dying, the doctor has suddenly become obsessed with learning the truth. He interrogates the mother, while callously ignoring her anguish: Could Petrov be the boy's father? Or what about Korovsky? As a doctor Tsvyetkov is able to approach his patient professionally with a mixture of detachment and compassion, but what if he is the father? That would be too much. He must feel that the weight of love and sorrow would crush him. Thus, he desperately searches for a new "truth."

DARKNESS

What is the appropriate use of social power in medicine? In "Darkness" (1887) a peasant accosts the district doctor and asks him to intervene on behalf of the peasant's imprisoned brother. The brother was drunk; he didn't mean any harm. The brother is poor and has a family to feed. Surely, the doctor will explain the situation and be able to get the fellow out of jail. The doctor withdraws in disgust. How ignorant these peasants are! They have no idea of how the world works. "There is nothing I can do," he tells the man.

There is nothing I can do.

The title of the story is "Darkness." What is the darkness at issue here? The ignorance of the peasant, whose faith in the doctor is irrational? In this view the doctor may represent the light of reason. It should be clear that he couldn't intervene in a matter of law. The man committed a crime. There is nothing to be done. Or is there? Perhaps "darkness" refers to the doctor—to his lack of vision, his inability to see the suffering that is going on around him. The Zemstvo doctor might view himself simply as a government functionary. Why put himself out for a peasant? Why get involved? And then, of course, the doctor could always raise the well-known bureaucratic argument: if I went out on the limb for your brother, I'd have to do it for everybody who asked. Where would I draw the line? I'll just mind my own business, thank you, and stay here in the dark.

Enemies

In this tale from 1887, Chekhov presents a physician who struggles to fulfill the ideals of his profession. Kirilov, whose child has just died of diphtheria, confronts a desperate landowner who wants to drag him out on a house call to see his wife who, the landowner is convinced, is seriously ill. Should the doctor abandon his own distraught wife and set aside his own grief to make this emergency call? He vacillates but eventually decides that professional duty comes first.

When Kirilov accompanies Abogin, they discover that the wife is not sick—rather, she has flown the coop! She had duped her husband, then used his absence to elope with her lover. Kirilov's passion surges. "Allow me to ask what is the meaning of this," he demands, his face livid with anger. The doctor spews forth his hatred for the wealthy gentry, people who lead lives of indolence while others spend their lives working for a living. "You look upon doctors and people generally who work and don't stink of perfume and prostitution as your menials." Abogin responds by reminding him that even the wealthy have feelings. "It is ungenerous," he says. "I am intensely unhappy myself."

However, Kirilov's heart has hardened against his enemy. The two men remain locked in separate worlds.

The Examining Magistrate

In "The Examining Magistrate" (1887), two professional men are driving through the country on their way to conduct an inquest. One of them, the examining magistrate, begins to tell the other, a doctor, that he knows many stories of mysterious deaths, deaths that presumably could not be explained by scientific inquiry. He goes on to tell the story of a young pregnant woman who was convinced that she would die shortly after giving birth. Indeed, despite the fact that she was apparently healthy, the woman died as she predicted.

Rather than accepting these events as evidence of mysterious powers, the doctor asks the magistrate a series of questions about the events—questions very analogous to clinical history taking. Given this new information, the doctor weighs the probabilities and then comes to a diagnosis. His explanation is convincing and thoroughly scientific. Unfortunately, this demonstration of the power of good clinical decision making has unintended consequences—for the woman in question was the magistrate's wife and the new "diagnosis" brings him great pain.

AN AWKWARD BUSINESS

In Chekhov's world physicians live uneasily at the interface of class conflict. Many intellectuals of the time idealized peasants and their simple lifestyle, believing that the poor are naturally good, kindhearted people, who are corrupted by civilization, especially by the brutal drudgery heaped on them by landowners. These intellectuals held a Rousseau-like view that the peasants (about 80 percent of the Russian population) were noble savages, whose good traits ought to be nourished and emulated. After his midlife religious conversion, Tolstoy, too, held this belief. In his later years, Tolstoy sometimes dressed in ragged clothes and worked the fields alongside his servants. This idealization of the peasantry carried with it a sense of class guilt. However, Chekhov, himself the grandson of serfs, held no such romantic belief. He was convinced that meanness and ignorance were deeply embedded in the society and could not be easily thrust aside. "Peasant blood flows through my veins," he wrote to Suvorin, "and you can't astonish me with peasant virtue" (to Suvorin, March 27, 1894).

In "An Awkward Business" (1888), Ovchinnikov is an overworked doctor in charge of a poorly staffed hospital. One morning on rounds, Dr. Ovchinnikov realizes that his incompetent assistant (*feldsher*) has a hangover and is not performing his job correctly. "You're not fit to be trusted," the doctor cries. In a fit of rage, he slugs the assistant, then runs out of the ward, but soon returns to complete rounds and see an additional forty-five patients in the clinic.

The assistant naturally fears for his job. He tries to apologize for his drunkenness, but Ovchinnikov, strangely, has begun to ruminate over his own guilt. He wonders how he, an educated person, could allow himself to lose control over the peccadilloes of an ignorant *feldsher*. Can his violence be justified? The doctor goes so far as to suggest that Smirinovsky ought to sue him for damages. "Let him sue me, I shan't defend myself, I was in the wrong, those who looked up to me will see that I was wrong." Ovchinnikov decides he has abased himself so much that he ought to resign from the hospital. Needless to say, his boss, the chairman of the hospital board, finds the whole affair a bit perplexing.

In "An Awkward Business" we see not only the class guilt motif, but also the modern theme of occupational stress—where small, everyday problems of practice gradually build to a great tide that overwhelms the protagonist. Medicine is ripe with opportunities for chronic stress, alienation, and burnout. Chekhov develops this theme further in later, more complex tales, such as "A Dreary Story" (1889) and "Ward No. 6" (1892). However, in this case, the distraught Dr. Ovchinnikov concludes, "Everything had fizzled out in a finale so banal."

THE PRINCESS

"The Princess" (1889) provides another example of class conflict. Mikhail Ivanovitch is an elderly widowed doctor who donates his time to a monastery, where he encounters his former employer, Princess Vera Gavrilovna. The cruel and imperious princess frequently visits the monastery, where she has her own comfortable apartment, and confesses her sins to the abbot. On this occasion she is feeling so virtuous that she asks the doctor to tell her the truth about her own shortcomings. At her insistence he ticks off a list of incidents that demonstrate her self-centeredness and contempt for peasants and retainers. The princess is astonished. My God, what is the world coming to? How can a mere physician speak to her like this? Mikhail Ivanovitch continues:

> For example, allow me to ask why did you dismiss me? For ten years I worked for your father and, afterwards, for you, honestly, without vacations or holidays. I gained the love of all for more than seventy miles around, and suddenly one fine day I am informed that I am no longer wanted. What for? I have no idea to this day. I, a doctor of medicine, a gentleman by birth, a student of the Moscow University, father of a family—am such a petty, insignificant insect that you can kick me out without explaining the reason!

Chekhov chooses not to end the story with this emotionally satisfying put-down but rather has the doctor return to apologize to the princess. "Forgive me, for God's sake," he says. "I was carried away by an evil, vindictive feeling and I talked . . . nonsense." What does this apology say about the man's character? Is it really a change of heart? It is interesting that the meeting takes place in a monastery, a setting that reminds us of the Christian belief that only God is justified in judging another person's heart. Mikhail Ivanovitch's apology seems to demonstrate his self-effacement or humility, a very important, but often neglected, virtue in medical practice.

A NERVOUS BREAKDOWN

In "A Nervous Breakdown" (1889) three young men decide to spend a night cruising the red-light district of Moscow. Mayer, a medical student, and Rybnikov, an artist, are old hands at enjoying the pleasures of S Street, but their friend Vassilyev, a law student, "knew nothing of fallen women except by hearsay and from books, and he had never in his life been in the houses in which they live." Vassilyev agrees to come along, but cringes in the background, and finds himself overwhelmed by the whores' tough, unrepentant attitude, and by the social inequities that led them to become prostitutes. He had imagined the women would gladly confess to any sympathetic ear. Instead, he discovers "on every face nothing but a blank expression of everyday vulgar boredom and complacency."

Vassilyev collapses with a nervous breakdown, crying, "My God, those women are alive!" As a future physician, Mayer approaches the situation from a cold, professional perspective. In essence, he diagnoses Vassilyev as being too thin-skinned and inexperienced. "One must take an objective view of things," Mayer says; one must suppress emotion and learn detachment. When the nervous symptoms persist, Vassilyev is taken to a psychiatrist, who reinforces this attitude. After all, the psychiatrist suggests, there is nothing you can do about prostitution. Toughen yourself, become more objective, and get on with your life.

Thus, Chekhov introduces the double-edged sword of objectivity. The ability to make systematic and clear observations is an important medical skill. In doing this, the physician cannot afford to be overwhelmed by emotion. Yet, if objectivity prevents us from recognizing others' feelings, we risk becoming cold and hardhearted. To use the words of Thomas Percival, the British Enlightenment physician who wrote the first modern book of medical ethics (1803), unless physicians view detachment as a serious professional risk and seek to cultivate "tender charity" in their professional relationships, they are vulnerable to "coldness of heart" and "moral insensibility."

WARD NO. 6

Dr. Ragin, the protagonist of "Ward No. 6" (1892), lives in a world of emotional numbness. In charge of a district hospital for twenty years, Ragin started out as an energetic doctor who made rounds every day, worked long hours in the clinic, and tried to keep up as well as he could with the latest scientific developments. However, time has eroded his vision. He now sees the "palpable futility" of medicine and has concluded that his efforts have made no difference. The hospital is poorly equipped and out-of-date. Social and economic forces beyond his control determine health and disease. In response, Ragin has retreated into a shell, a world without passion, a place of solitude with few human contacts. While an assistant actually performs his job at the hospital, Ragin sits in his study and reads.

Heavy demands and poor working conditions contribute to Ragin's predicament, but he faces a deeper problem as well. Something is missing. Is his sense of futility really a consequence of medical practice? Many of Chekhov's characters suffer from a lack of self-knowledge, wandering through their lives relying on one form of self-deception after another, and often causing great pain to other people. Ragin is like that. When he was younger, he meant well and committed himself to noble ideals. But in the long run, the center didn't hold, and he never "found" himself. Ragin experiences this failure as emotional numbness.

At one point Ragin visits the mental ward (Ward No. 6), where he meets Ivan Gromov, a brilliant paranoid who embraces life passionately. The passion attracts Ragin like a moth to the flame. Ragin yearns to feel something, anything, even to experience suffering, rather than to remain suspended in his emotionless cocoon. He develops an obsession that only the experience of suffering can save him. This obsession makes him even more dysfunctional, a situation the regional authorities exploit by firing him and, ultimately, committing him to the mental ward. Once Ragin becomes a patient, a "nobody," his protective cocoon disappears, and for a brief moment the doctor achieves his elusive goal—he suffers.

THE GRASSHOPPER

"The Grasshopper" (1982) depicts Dr. Dymov standing in the wings, devoting his energies to medical practice and research. He tends to fade into the woodwork, while at center stage is Olga, Dymov's wife, whose passion is the gay, artistic life her staid husband is unable to provide for her. However, Olga discovers a new lease on romance with Ryabovsky, a colorful landscape artist, who takes her on a cruise and promises her nothing. After Olga returns from the cruise, Dymov forgives her infidelity, but even his ability to forgive proves in Olga's eyes to be another strike against the poor slob. Dymov's devotion drives her up the wall.

Chekhov based this story on the real-life love affair of his good friend Isaak Levitan, a well-known married painter, with Lika Mizinova, a young unmarried teacher who was, more or less, on the rebound from her unrequited passion for the author himself. The character of the doctor/husband clearly has its roots in Dr. Chekhov, visualized in the story as a dedicated and disciplined professional who could spare no time for frivolous romance.

Dymov's death turns the tables, as he assumes the role of a martyr. Was his death the result of a technical error? Did Olga's infidelity play a role, perhaps in distracting him as he was aspirating pus from the throat of a diphtheria patient? Or might Dymov have deliberately aspirated the material, realizing that the subsequent infection would likely cause his death? In any case, Olga at last realizes that her husband was indeed a hero.

THE HEAD GARDENER'S STORY

In "The Head Gardener's Story" (1894), the doctor leaves the stage before the play begins. Here he is victim, rather than protagonist. Was Dr. Thomson killed in a freak accident, or by malevolent design? One thing is sure; he was the best doctor anyone in town had ever known. "They were glad that God had sent them at last a man who could heal diseases, and were proud that such a remarkable man was living in their town." Thomson was a saint: "He loved them like children, and did not spare himself for them. He was himself ill with consumption, he had a cough, but when he was summoned to the sick he forgot his own illness, he did not spare himself and, gasping for breath, climbed up the hills, however high they may be." As it turns out, Thomson suffers the fate of many saints before him.

"The Head Gardener's Story" might be an allegory about the conflict between science and faith, or between reason and the irrational forces that govern much of human life. The villagers cling to their blind faith in human goodness, despite persuasive evidence that evil has occurred. Although they acknowledge the existence of the evidence, they interpret it in light of their preconceived theories.

This story is reminiscent of the great intellectual conflicts of the Renaissance. Take, for example, the medieval penchant of accounting for new observations about the movement of the planets by making ad hoc changes to the Ptolemaic theory that the earth is the center of the universe. The Ptolemaic system developed an array of messy loops and epicycles to keep it faithfully in place. It took Copernicus to "see" the evidence in a new way, move the sun to the center, and restore simplicity to the model. Similarly, in 1542 Vesalius demonstrated that the septum dividing the human heart into left and right ventricles is solid. The pores or openings predicated by Galen simply do not exist. Galenic physiology, which had held sway for thirteen hundred years, needed those pores to explain how blood could pass from the right side of the heart to the left. The orthodoxy was so entrenched that for nearly one hundred years most observers tried to reconcile observation with theory by explaining away Vesalius's observations (e.g., the pores closed after death, thus obviating them in the cadaver). Only in 1628 did William Harvey demonstrate that Vesalius was correct by devising an elegant new theory of his own—the theory that blood circulates, rather than waxing and waning like the tides.

It is interesting indeed that Dr. Chekhov chose a practicing physician to serve as a symbol of both science and saintliness.

IONITCH

"Ionitch" (1898) depicts the deconstruction of Dr. Startsev, a young physician who at the outset has just completed his medical training. When he arrives at his new station, the wealthy Turkin family invites him to dinner. There, he meets their daughter Ykaterina who teases the infatuated Startsev but then runs off to Moscow to become a professional pianist. In this way she hopes to escape her "empty, futile existence." Initially, the jilted lover is bitter, but he gradually regains his composure, dives into his work, and eventually becomes a wealthy and corpulent practitioner.

"Ionitch" traces the progressive change that may occur in a physician who finds that medical affluence is more to his or her liking than the emotionally and physically difficult path of caring for patients. Initially, we glimpse Startsev as young and relatively unformed. His abortive romance results in a conscious decision to harden himself and turn away from the affective world. To avoid getting hurt a second time, he will never again become emotionally involved. Although "Ionitch" places this change in a romantic context, the course seems similar to that of a lifetime of medical detachment, in which the doctor gradually comes to look on feelings as his enemy. As with Mayer in "A Nervous Breakdown," we confront Startsev's coldness of heart, in his case a glacial coldness.

A DOCTOR'S VISIT

In "A Doctor's Visit" (1898) a young doctor makes a house call at the behest of his boss, the professor of medicine in Moscow. It is a thankless task—the daughter of a wealthy factory owner is having another attack of palpitations, insomnia, and nervousness. The doctor, whose name is Korolyov, quickly ascertains that the "poor, destitute creature" suffers from no identifiable disease. Her heart is intact— or at least, her physical heart.

Her metaphorical heart is quite another matter. Korolyov agrees to stay for supper and spend the night. During the evening, as he meanders around the factory buildings, he undergoes an epiphany, experiencing a flash of insight into the connection between the patient's illness and the oppressive environment in which she lives. "It is just like being in prison," he observes. While the factory workers are caught in a heartless, grinding machine of poverty, the owners and supervisors are also caught in the same malevolent system, which makes them mean and insensitive.

The young man's sudden perception of emotional and spiritual malaise leads him to look at his patient differently. At first Korolyov approached her with detached concern, a standard mixture of openness and professional reserve. After his insight, Korolyov views her through the lens of compassionate solidarity. He has tuned in and become sensitive to her feelings, as well as to her heart sounds. In turn, she responds to his empathy with self-revelation. She reveals that, in fact, she suffers from "no illness," but rather is "weary and frightened" of life. Although Korolyov doesn't prescribe a treatment, it seems that the patient has benefited from his presence, as exemplified by her rising the next morning and wearing a white dress with a flower.

A Selected Chronology for Chekhov's Doctors

1881–1884
Triletsky, *Platonov* (play)
Shelestov, "Intrigues"*
The Pharmacist, "At the Pharmacy"
The Doctor, "Perpetuum Mobile"

1885
Marfa Petrovna Petchonkin, "Malingerers" (homeopathic physician)*
Stepan Lukitch, "The Looking-Glass"

1886
Tsvyetkov, "The Doctor"*
Vera, "Excellent People"*
Stepan Klotchkov, "Anyuta"*
Koshelkov, "A Work of Art"

1887
The Zemstvo Doctor, "Darkness"*
Kirilov, "Enemies"*
The District Doctor, "The Examining Magistrate"*

1888
Ovchinnikov, "An Awkward Business"*
The Doctor, "Lights"

1889
Lvov, *Ivanov* (play)
Mikhail Ivanovitch, "The Princess"*
Mayer, "A Nervous Breakdown"*
Nikolai Stepanovich, "A Boring Story"

1891
Samoylenko, "The Duel"

1892
Osip Dymov, "The Grasshopper"*
Ragin, "Ward No. 6"*
Sobol, "The Wife"

1894
Thomson, "The Head Gardener's Story"*

1895
Dorn, *The Sea Gull* (play)

1896
Astrov, *Uncle Vanya* (play)
Blagovo, "My Life"

1897
Neshtchapov, "At Home"

1898
Korolyov, "A Doctor's Visit"*
Startsev, "Ionitch"*
Ivan Ivanovitch Tchimsha-Himalaisky, "Gooseberries," "The Man in a Case," and
    "About Love" (veterinary surgeon)

1899
Starchenko, "On Official Business"

1900
Chebutykin, *The Three Sisters* (play)

*Stories included in this collection.

Sources

The sources of the following stories are from *The Tales of Chekhov* in thirteen volumes, translated by Constance Garnett, published by Ecco Press, New York, 1984–1986:

"Malingerers" *The Schoolmaster and Other Stories,*
vol. 11. 269–74

"Excellent People" *The Duel and Other Stories,*
vol. 2, 175–91

"Anyuta" *The Darling and Other Stories,*
vol. 1, 85–91

"Darkness" *The Horse-Stealers and Other Stories,*
vol. 10, 171–76

"Enemies" *The Schoolmaster and Other Stories,*
vol. 11, 15–34

"The Examining Magistrate" *The Schoolmaster and Other Stories,*
vol. 11, 37–44

"The Princess" *The Duel and Other Stories,*
vol. 2, 293–312

"A Nervous Breakdown" *The Schoolmistress and Other Stories,*
vol. 9, 17–53

"Ward No. 6" *The Horse-Stealers and Other Stories,*
vol. 10, 29–109

"The Grasshopper" *The Wife and Other Stories,*
vol. 5, 89–127

"The Head Gardener's Story" *The Schoolmistress and Other Stories,*
vol. 9, 267–76

"Ionitch" *The Lady with the Dog and Other Stories,*
vol. 3, 65–92

"A Doctor's Visit" *The Lady with the Dog and Other Stories,*
vol. 3, 31–48

The sources of other stories in this collection are as follows:

"Intrigues"	*The Undiscovered Chekhov. Forty-three New Stories.* Trans. Peter Constantine. New York, Seven Stories Press, 1999. 165–72.
"The Doctor"	*Anton Chekhov. Early Short Stories 1883–1888.* Ed. Shelby Foote. New York, Trans. Constance Garnett. Modern Library Edition, 1999. 408–13.
"An Awkward Business"	*The Unknown Chekhov. Stories and Other Writings.* Trans. Avtahm Yarmolinsky. New York, Ecco Press, 1987. 137–60.

Selected Bibliography

❧

Callow, Phillip. *Chekhov: The Hidden Ground.* Chicago: Ivan R. Dee, 1998.

Chekhov, Anton. *A Journey to Sakhalin.* Trans. Brian Reeve. Cambridge: Ian Faulkner, 1993.

———. *Letters of Anton Chekhov.* Ed. Simon Karlinsky. Trans. Michael Henry Heim. New York: Harper & Row, 1973.

Coope, John. *Doctor Chekhov. A Study in Literature and Medicine.* Chale, Isle of Wight: Cross, 1997.

Jackson, Robert Louis, ed. *Reading Chekhov's Text.* Evanston, Ill.: Northwestern Univ. Press, 1993

Johnson, Ronald L. *Anton Chekhov: A Study of the Short Fiction,* New York: Twayne, 1993.

Kataev. Vladimir. *If Only We Could Know. An Interpretation of Chekhov.* Chicago, Ill.: Ivan R. Dee, 2002

Malcolm, Janet. *Reading Chekhov. A Critical Journey.* New York: Random House, 2001.

Pritchett, V. S. *Chekhov: A Spirit Set Free.* New York: Random House, 1988

Rayfield, Donald. *Anton Chekhov. A Life.* New York: Henry Holt, 1997.

———. *Understanding Chekhov. A Critical Study of Chekhov's Prose and Drama.* Madison: Univ. of Wisconsin Press, 1999.

Simmons, Ernest R. *Chekhov. A Biography.* Boston: Little, Brown, & Co., 1962.

Troyat, Henri. *Chekhov.* New York: E. P. Dutton, 1986.